NEXT-LEVEL METABOLISM

NEXT LEVEL METABOLISM

THE ART & SCIENCE
of METABOLIC MASTERY

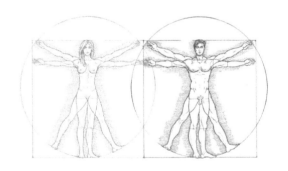

DR. JADE TETA

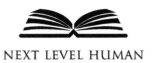

NEXT LEVEL HUMAN

NEXT-LEVEL METABOLISM
The Art and Science of Metabolic Mastery

ISBN   978-1-5445-2491-7   *Hardcover*
           978-1-5445-2490-0   *Paperback*
           978-1-5445-2489-4   *Ebook*

To the artist-scientists who stand on the edge of the known and leap courageously into the unknown. Their creative courage, their willingness to be wrong, and their unyielding commitment to evidence are what make all progress possible. This book is for them. Thank you for your work and for inspiring me to attempt the same.

CONTENTS

INTRODUCTION

You might think you know everything there is to know about metabolism. If you work in the health and wellness field, you've likely done your fair share of research on the topic, yet you still might be struggling to make sense of the overload of conflicting information you've come across. Or maybe you're just someone who loves fitness and by now, you might think no outside source could possibly teach you about mastering your own metabolism because no one understands your unique physiology better than you.

No matter how much you think you do or don't know about it, I'm here to tell you, *metabolism is not exactly what you may think it is.*

Most of what we all think we know about metabolism is based on outdated information that's long been widely accepted—until now. Science is an ongoing process, one that is constantly emerging and evolving as we get closer and closer to understanding ourselves and the world around us. New thinking continues to replace old ideas, resulting in a long list of metabolism dos and don'ts that have come and gone over the last few decades. First, we were told we should eliminate fat. Next, it was all about ditching the carbs. Throughout, we were convinced nothing mattered but counting calories. After that, hormones got the spotlight. Year after year, no magic one-size-fits-all diet ever worked because the thinking behind them was always incomplete. That's because the truth is, metabolism is about all of those things—nutrition, exercise, calories, and hormones—and how they work together will look different for *every single individual human being*.

Learning to understand your unique metabolism is like learning to play an instrument or speak a different language. It takes time. You're not going to learn it from a recipe book or a meal plan or by watching a documentary or listening to a podcast.

You won't master it by adhering to one outdated school of thought and remaining mentally rigid, because there is no place for bias or dogma when it comes to metabolism. In fact, there is only one rule that you need to know: *Do what works for you.*

You cannot outsource this responsibility. To master your metabolism, you must go through a discovery process of what works and what doesn't and then create a diet *for you by you.* This book is an attempt to teach you how to do just that. No one can know your metabolism as well as you do, and as soon as you learn how to listen to it and interpret what it's telling you, you can finally get off the weight-loss roller coaster you've likely been riding most of your life.

One thing you should know before you get started: this book is not a diet book. If you are hoping to find meal plans, recipes, workouts, and prescriptions for exactly what to do, you are in the wrong place. That attitude is the very reason people fail again and again.

I refuse to play that same tired game. If you want to learn how to figure it out for yourself—the only way it will ever and has ever worked—then you are in the right place. Otherwise, there are a million other "diet books" out there that claim to teach the holy grail of body change. This book teaches you how to do that for yourself.

You should also know that I have purposely repeated concepts throughout the book. Don't be surprised if some passages feel like a repeat of something you have already read. I did this on purpose because I am a big believer in repetition of concepts, especially when it comes to a subject matter as complex as metabolism.

Finally, I hope you understand this book is a detailed dive into the existing body of scientific literature and my clinical experience. What that means is that we know very little about metabolism. This work is part art and part science, the art being my clinical experience and best educated guesses and the science being the research studies and their current consensus. Rest assured that some of this material will be upgraded in future years and decades. Some of it may be outright wrong. That's the nature of this field. We are always upgrading our understandings and revising what we once thought. My hope with this work is to give you a solid base in both the art and the science so you can begin evolving your understanding as you practice the art and the science advances.

THE ULTIMATE BAROMETER

Every person's metabolism has one quality in common: it is never static. Metabolism is not like a calculator, prepared to spit out the same answer no matter how often you input the equation. It's more like a barometer and a thermostat, surveying its surroundings and always changing its response based on the conditions to which it's exposed. It's adaptive and reactive, always measuring, sensing, assessing, then developing the appropriate response. It does this every second of every day, never taking a break, never missing a single thing.

As it does this, it's constantly striving for balance, all the while determining how hungry you are, what you're craving, how much energy you have, what kind of mood you're in, and how well you sleep.

The fact that metabolism is never static means that to master it, you must become comfortable with change. The way you work with your metabolism will evolve as you move through your life, and this book will also prepare you for such situations. Illness, stress, pregnancy, menopause, andropause, and aging are just a few things that can impact metabolism. You will have to learn to adapt to such changes and manage the stress they are capable of creating.

The process is not about some one-time thing someone can try, then run back to their old way of life, which is what most dieters do. The most hidden, insidious cause of obesity and weight gain in the first place is dieting, which is nothing more than starvation from your metabolism's perspective. When it finds itself in that place, it is going to do everything it can to recoup energy, which only makes it harder to lose fat in the long run. Here are just a few stats to illustrate just how bleak the results of traditional "dieting" can be:

- Ninety-five percent of people who lose weight on the standard eat less, exercise more way of dieting end up regaining it all back within a year.
- Sixty-six percent end up fatter.

- Within two years, 97 percent have gained it all back.
- Within three years, almost every single person has regained it all and then some.[1]

The reason for the relapse is simple: metabolism is constantly adapting. It is never not paying attention. So when you allow yourself to keep doing the same thing day in and day out for an extended period of time, your metabolism is literally laughing at you. It's saying, "What the hell is wrong with you? I already have adapted. Time to switch things up!" It's why your approach to losing the weight has to be different than your approach to maintaining your weight.

It's why you must alter your approach as you age. Most importantly, it's why you have to learn to speak the language of metabolism so you always know exactly what it's trying to tell you.

Metabolism's one job is to keep us alive long enough to reproduce. It's always making sure we have enough fuel to support reproduction (this is why female metabolism is more sensitive and refined than male metabolism—much more on this later). So what does metabolism perpetually respond to? One thing and one thing only: stress, meaning anything that knocks metabolism out of balance. Not all stress is bad—a small amount that only rattles metabolism slightly can help it adapt and become stronger. This short-lived stress, known as eustress or hormetic stress, can be highly beneficial. However, any stress that knocks metabolism too far out of balance for too long will cause it to respond and react too intensely.

The most significant stress the metabolism encountered throughout its evolution is starvation. When it senses starvation, the metabolism activates all of the behaviors that can save us from it, including increased hunger and cravings. Starvation also wreaks havoc with your energy because if you don't have enough fuel, the best thing for your metabolism is to sit still, do nothing, and conserve its energy. At the same time, it also wants to motivate you to go out and find food. This causes your energy to be unpredictable and unstable. One minute you're wired, motivated, and focused, and the next you're drained, foggy-headed, and can think of nothing but sleep. Basically, you're a mess, and a hungry one at that.

All of these factors constantly tell you whether your metabolism is balanced and how it functions when under stress. If you want to understand how to take mastery of your metabolism to the next level, you need to know what it's designed to do first, then learn to decipher all the messages it's constantly sending you.

MY METABOLISM WAKE-UP CALL

Metabolism has always been on my radar, ever since my early days of playing sports when I first realized how proper nutrition was capable of elevating my performance. The relationship fascinated me and sent me digging deeper into biochemistry. I started training others and writing programs for them to follow to reach maximum results. I went on to study biochemistry in college, and medical school seemed to be the next logical step. However, when I started to look into the curriculum, I was disappointed to see how it lacked adequate training in diet and exercise. I knew I didn't want to just prescribe drugs and perform surgery—not that there's anything wrong with drugs and surgery—but I already knew the power of diet and exercise, and I was certain it was what I wanted my life to be about. Fortunately, I found a program centered on functional medicine. I would earn a doctorate in naturopathic medicine, a little-known field of study at the time aimed at primary care doctors who wanted to specialize in lifestyle medicine.

Back then, no one knew alternative and complementary medicine would eventually become mainstream, and when I announced I was enrolling in this program, people were quick to dissuade me. They told me it was witchcraft, too niche, certainly not a field in which to make a living. But I knew I wanted to teach health and fitness, and this was how I wanted to do it.

When I was getting my medical degree, I still wanted to be in the gym working with people. I specialized in weight loss and quickly discovered that women, compared to men, were far more proactive and engaged in their health and fitness endeavors. As a result, the vast majority of people I worked with were female. But not all of my clients were getting the results I expected them to. It didn't take long for me to realize there was one big problem: *me*. Late-twenties Jade was not the informed, patient person capable of seeing everyone as a unique individual that I hope I am today. I was ignorant, arrogant, and totally convinced that the one way I thought you should do things was the only way to do it. At that time, I was pushing low-carb diets and high-intensity interval training for *every single person who came to me*. That's what worked for me and my friends at the gym. That was what new research was touting. I was totally confused when I found this approach wasn't working for all people. In fact, it was failing for many of my female clients, most especially my more mature female clientele.

At the time, I assumed they were just being lazy, gluttonous even. I figured it had to be an issue of compliance. Maybe they were not doing what I had prescribed? Turned out their cookie consumption was not the issue—my cookie-cutter approach to helping them was.

Luckily (albeit embarrassingly at the time), one woman put me in my place. Once when I was training with her and pushing her really hard, she suddenly burst into tears. This threw me for a loop—the gym wasn't for crying. What the heck was going on?

She was quick to tell me.

"What the hell is wrong with you?" she said through sobs. "I am not a young athlete. I am not training to compete. *I am not some young male bodybuilder.*"

Then she asked the question that would change my approach to metabolism forever: "How on earth can you help me if you don't even understand who I am and how my body works?"

That moment was such a gift. She couldn't have been more right. I realized then that each person has a unique physiology and psychology, and when you don't take that into account, you are guaranteed to fail. I started learning everything I could about hormones, how they affect men and women differently, how to achieve balance, and how they work with metabolism. I started to see metabolism as a biological thermostat, capable of adapting and changing depending on how you use it.

This thinking led me to develop the program I use now to help people achieve real, lasting, sustainable results. I've been able to help countless people over the course of the last thirty years, including my own mother who, until I was able to apply this new understanding to a program I developed specifically for her, had struggled with weight loss during and after menopause. What worked for her was not anything I previously would have considered. Her experience solidified in me an understanding that metabolic expression is like a fingerprint and is different for every single human being on this planet.

Had I continued to be closed-minded, I would have missed the opportunity to help her and so many others.

To date, I've written several other books on the subject, contributed to textbooks, and lectured to doctors, nutritionists, and chiropractors worldwide. This book is the culmination of that knowledge and experience. It is a comprehensive overview of everything I know about metabolism today. I present this information to you with the understanding that science is always emerging, and that will change our understanding of how our bodies work. But knowing what we do know now, I can say with great confidence that the key to taking your metabolism to the next level is being humble enough to know you are not in charge. Your metabolism is directing the show—it's up to you to learn the script. It is no longer appropriate to study what the gurus, diet books, blogs, podcasts, documentaries, and popular media are telling you, and that includes me. Instead, I want to help you start studying yourself. No one can know your body as well as you can. You are the only one who matters here. It's time to start the journey of self-discovery by determining your own metabolic processes instead of outsourcing that job to someone else. That's what I hope this book does for you. Let's get started.

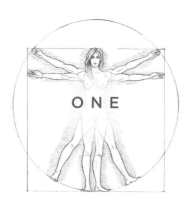

THE NEW SCIENCE OF METABOLISM

here's one complaint I have become nearly sick of hearing. People say it all the time. You likely hear it too if you work in the health and wellness field. Maybe it's something you've said to yourself again and again, your frustration building every time the thought nags at your mind. The most common gripe among people trying and failing to lose weight is, "I'm doing everything right, but I'm still not getting results."

As tempting as it might be to use a claim like this to absolve ourselves of any blame for our lack of progress, the truth is simple: *If you're doing everything right and not getting results, then you're not doing everything right.*

Most likely, the reason you're not doing everything right is that you're outsourcing your metabolism to other people. You're expecting your favorite podcaster or the latest diet book or some guy named Jade to give you a one-size-fits-all solution to making your metabolism yield to your wants. You think you can do the same thing your friend did and get the same results. You're treating your metabolism like a video game you can turn on whenever you want and play on your terms. *That's not how any of this works.* By denying you any real results, your metabolism is basically grabbing you by the shirt collar and screaming, "You better figure me out because if you don't, there is no way I am ever going to work with you!"

The new science of metabolism is rooted in the idea that everyone is uniquely different. No two people have the same metabolism working in exactly the same way. Therefore, no two people are going to get results from the same single approach. Furthermore, each person's metabolism always has a reason for doing whatever it is doing at any given moment in time. It never acts randomly; it's never unprovoked. And if it seems as if your metabolism is acting against you rather than with you, I can promise you it is also desperately trying to tell you why.

Your metabolism is always talking to you, but before you can ever begin to interpret its message, you first have to understand its language. The metabolism doesn't speak English; it speaks metabolism. If you hope to understand it, you are going to need to learn how to hear it. When it comes to deciphering the language of metabolism, you need to become acquainted with the three rules governing its behavior. I call them the three laws of metabolism.

LAW #1:
THE LAW OF METABOLIC FLEXIBILITY

It might seem logical to assume a fast metabolism is ideal, but the truth is, you don't want a fast metabolism—you want a *flexible* metabolism. The reasoning is simple: if you speed up metabolism, you also speed up hunger and cravings. A flexible metabolism, however, doesn't let a lack of food send it straight into starvation behaviors. You want a metabolism that can adapt to the environmental stresses and strains it will experience.

Your metabolism should be like a thick rubber band you can pull and stretch and turn every single way. However, the more you do the traditional weight loss approach of eat less, exercise more (which I abbreviate as ELEM), the more your metabolism becomes like one of those skinny, frayed bands that break as soon as you pull them. ELEM creates an extreme calorie gap, which is the difference in the amount of energy you're taking in and the amount of energy you're putting out. The longer you try to stay in that gap, the more stress you're putting on your metabolism. What does the stress barometer do to compensate? It increases hunger and cravings and makes energy unstable. And that's not the worst of it. It also downregulates your resting metabolic rate. This is a natural protective mechanism against hunger. Some research suggests an average decline of 100 calories resting energy use.[2] However, certain individuals can see resting metabolic rates decline by over 300 calories daily. Still others may see no change.

So you go on an ELEM diet, bust your butt to create a 300-calorie deficit, work like crazy to stay on that diet, and your metabolism rewards you by ramping up hunger and wiping out energy.

The result? *No results.*

ELEM puts you in a tug-of-war with your metabolism. You pull on it, it pulls back; you pull again, it pulls back even harder until it literally yanks you off your feet. Do you know the only way to win a tug-of-war match against a stronger opponent? When they pull, you let go of the rope. In this case, that means realizing ELEM can no longer be the only solution you have.

If you keep doing ELEM for long periods of time, your metabolism becomes more and more rigid until you make some real changes to get it back to its normally flexible state.

Metabolic compensation is also the reason why the casts of *Biggest Loser* aren't lining up to do reunion shows. Most of those people not only gained back all the weight they lost, but they also threw their metabolism out of whack. A study of some of the contestants six years after their participation showed most have metabolic derangements that make it harder for them to achieve and maintain weight loss.[3] The good news, however, is that you can't ever "break" your metabolism. Metabolism will always do whatever it naturally does. You can, however, reverse any damage you might have done by adhering to the new science.

Metabolic Compensation and Multitasking

To fully appreciate how metabolism functions, you must understand two metabolic behaviors: metabolic compensation and metabolic multitasking. Metabolic compensation is relatively straightforward but has several elements to it. It is exactly what it sounds like: when the metabolism is confronted with stress in the outside world (temperature challenges, food shortages, threats to safety, exercise excess, etc.), it will institute its survival software and "compensate" in an attempt to regain balance. In essence, it is trying to mitigate extreme calorie imbalances and recoup any large energy losses.

For someone who is trying to lose body fat, this is an especially important process to understand. Metabolism acts like one big, sophisticated stress barometer, and a gap in the amount of energy you take in from food and the amount of energy you burn through activity is a major source of such stress. The wider that gap becomes, the more pressure the metabolic barometer registers. The energy gap widens and the metabolism reacts, which is what I call metabolic compensation.

There are several ways the metabolism begins to compensate, and none of them are helpful if you want to attain and maintain fat loss. Adaptive thermogenesis is the term used in research to describe a drop in metabolic rate to help mitigate against prolonged energy disturbances. Metabolism has several elements. Resting energy expenditure or REE (also called resting metabolic rate or RMR) is the number of calories the metabolism is burning at rest. REE is often used interchangeably with the basal metabolic rate or BMR, but they are slightly different. BMR is the amount of energy the metabolism burns when you are at rest first thing in the morning on a completely empty stomach (twelve hours of fasting) lying still in the dark. In other words, BMR is a slightly more stringent measurement than REE. But for the purposes of most discussions on metabolism, REE and BMR are considered synonymous unless you are a metabolism researcher. Basically, they represent the amount of energy you would need if you were to lie in your bed all day and do nothing else. Your metabolism uses a large amount of energy just to keep you alive, and REE and BMR are measures that try to quantify this minimum energy use.

BMR accounts for about 60–70 percent of metabolic energy use and is regulated largely by things outside of your immediate conscious control, such as the amount and activity of hormones like leptin, thyroid, estrogen, and testosterone. Immune regulation is also a sizable component of the amount of energy the metabolism uses at rest. Research estimates that an activated immune system can use 25–30 percent of BMR. Like the brain, the immune system adjusts the metabolism's energy priorities.

The brain and the immune system are also peculiar in the way they access the energy they need. Neither the brain nor the immune system requires insulin to access glucose. In fact, this may be one previously underappreciated aspect of insulin resistance. The brain (via control of stress hormones) and the immune system (through the release of inflammatory cytokines) can induce insulin resistance in other tissues. In the case of the brain, sympathetic neurons directly inhibit insulin release and peripheral hormones like cortisol antagonize the action of insulin at other tissues.

The immune system uses insulin in a different way. Like the brain, the immune system does not need insulin for its fuel needs; instead, it uses insulin as a growth promoter. Researchers have shown that immune cells are less numerous and less active when their insulin receptors are compromised.[4] This may be a "backdoor mechanism" the metabolism uses to free up glucose to the two systems most critical for its survival (the brain and immune system), while decreasing glucose use in all other tissues.

I realize this is complex biochemistry, but an understanding of the way the metabolism handles stress is essential. Stress to the metabolism includes infections, injury, and extreme gaps between energy intake and output.

When the metabolism is under assault from severe or prolonged calorie deficits induced by eating less and exercising more, it alters these metabolic hormones to bring the metabolic rate down. This is why the calorie levels predicted by weight loss equations are never accurate—they are trying to match a moving metabolic target.

It is important to address a few common objections related to reductions in resting energy use. Some argue that when a person loses weight, the number of calories they will burn is reduced. Obviously, if you have less body tissue, you will burn fewer calories. That's absolutely true; however, studies show that reductions in BMR are much greater than would be predicted based on weight loss alone.[5] In other words, a person who diets to 180 pounds will be burning fewer calories than if they were that same weight without dieting. Something about dieting adjusts the metabolic thermostat downward.

The body of research hints that approximately 5 percent of that downward reduction can last a very long time, perhaps permanently. Some researchers still debate the degree of this metabolic slowdown and whether it exists at all, pointing out that individuals measured in an isocaloric state don't show this effect, only those in a current hypocaloric state do.[6] This is a point of clarification we need to leave to future studies. At the time of this book, there is no consensus.

Another common belief is that BMR can be changed significantly with increased muscle mass. However, research shows there is only a six to thirty extra calorie burn with each pound of muscle (not a big difference-maker). Extra muscle makes its greatest contribution when it is moving, but metabolic compensation has an insidious effect there as well.

A final note on adaptive thermogenesis: it does work in the other direction. When the calorie gap moves from eating less and exercising more to exercising less and eating more, the metabolism will adjust its metabolic thermostat upward to dissipate some of the excess energy. That's the good news. The bad news is, this metabolic upregulation is less robust and responsive than the metabolic downregulation that occurs with dieting. This tells us something important about metabolism. In the evolution of human metabolism, metabolic compensation was more important to guard against starvation as compared to overfeeding. Our physiology has not had to deal with overcompensation for most of its existence.

In addition to reducing the BMR, the metabolism also compensates by reducing another component of metabolic output called NEAT. NEAT is an abbreviation for non-exercise activity thermogenesis, basically a fancy term for activities of daily living. When you go get the mail, walk up steps, brush your teeth, walk from your car to the store, have sex, do the laundry, walk the dog, fidget, or toss and turn in your sleep, NEAT is happening. The amount of energy burn accumulated through NEAT is one of the elements most underappreciated by dieters. NEAT makes up 15–20 percent of total daily energy burn. In comparison, the amount of energy burned through exercise (abbreviated EAT in research, exercise-associated thermogenesis) is only about 5 percent. This is one reason why casual walking (NEAT) *may* make a more significant contribution to weight loss than formal exercise

(EAT). It is also why NEAT and EAT (moving and exercise) need to be considered as separate things. *Exercise* is movement that is planned and structured, whereas activity of daily living (i.e., movement) is not. In this book, I will use "movement" as the word for NEAT and "exercise" as a word for EAT. Be sure to keep those distinctions in mind as you continue reading.

CONTRIBUTIONS TO ENERGY METABOLISM

Total daily energy expenditure (TDEE) is made up of two parts:

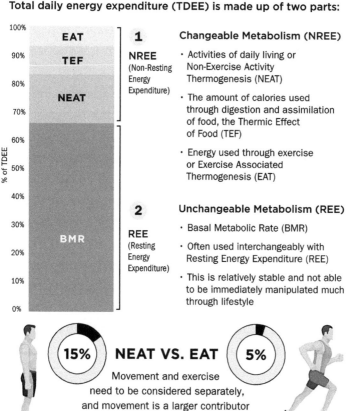

1 Changeable Metabolism (NREE)

NREE (Non-Resting Energy Expenditure)

- Activities of daily living or Non-Exercise Activity Thermogenesis (NEAT)
- The amount of calories used through digestion and assimilation of food, the Thermic Effect of Food (TEF)
- Energy used through exercise or Exercise Associated Thermogenesis (EAT)

2 Unchangeable Metabolism (REE)

REE (Resting Energy Expenditure)

- Basal Metabolic Rate (BMR)
- Often used interchangeably with Resting Energy Expenditure (REE)
- This is relatively stable and not able to be immediately manipulated much through lifestyle

15% NEAT VS. EAT 5%

Movement and exercise need to be considered separately, and movement is a larger contributor to energy use compared to exercise. (15% vs 5%)

You need to both move and exercise, but ultimately, movement may be more important. If I had to choose, I would rather you institute a walking program than an exercise program, and as you read further in this book, you'll understand exactly why.

Not only does the metabolism compensate by reducing resting metabolic rate, it also compensates by changing NEAT and EAT. To make up the calorie gap created with eating less and exercising more, the body spontaneously and unconsciously reduces the amount of NEAT it does. Even fidgeting and movements in sleep may be subconsciously reduced. Motivation to just get up and move also declines. This is another reason it is crucial to focus on moving over exercising.

The compensations against exercise-associated calorie burn are especially interesting. Most people think the energy they burn when they exercise is additive in nature. If you normally burn 2,000 calories at rest, then go for a 300-calorie run, you likely assume you burned 2,300 calories total. In fact, metabolic compensation causes the energy burned from exercise to be constrained. Whereas you may normally burn 300 calories on that run, a severe or prolonged calorie gap produced by eating less and exercising more reduces that calorie burn so that other metabolic parameters are reduced by 200–250 calories (the exact amount of reduction is debatable, so these numbers are just to illustrate the point). It's like trying to drive your car with the parking brake on—the car might move, but it is going much slower than it normally would.

This "constrained" metabolic response is not immediate but rather kicks in after several weeks or months of continuous exercise. Research has not yet determined if certain types of exercise

access to fresh produce. Or you might live in a food desert where the only place to shop for food is the nearest gas station. Your specific scenario is inevitably going to impact the approach you take to diet and exercise.

The law of metabolic individuality says all of these factors matter more than a little bit—they influence everything about how and why your metabolism does what it does. You must take each into consideration when engineering the approach that is going to work for you. Bruce Lee once said, we all must "absorb what is useful, discard what is useless, and add what is specifically your own." The same is true for creating the diet and exercise program that will work best for you. You have to honor your own uniqueness; otherwise, you have no chance of sustainable success.

When you cater your approach to your unique self, the seemingly impossible becomes very doable. My client Dale is a perfect example of this. Dale was a long-haul truck driver who was thirty pounds overweight and diabetic when his wife forced him to come to see me. "Look," he said the minute I met him, "I don't really want to be here. I am not into this natural food stuff." His main food sources, he told me, were truck stops, gas stations, and greasy spoons. I knew his unique physiology given his family history and current diabetes. I got a sense of his psychological tendencies, too. He was a simple guy, a hard worker who dealt with the stress of his job by enjoying food, keeping things convenient, and not worrying about too much else. His preferences and practical circumstances were crystal clear. It would have been ridiculous to assume he was going to go from an overweight diabetic living off fast food to a natural food enthusiast living off organic kale and wild-caught salmon.

THE 4Ps OF METABOLIC INDIVIDUALITY

Each human is as different on the inside biochemically as they are on the outside physically. We are each unique in our physiology, psychology, personal preferences, and practical circumstances. Any lifestyle intervention must account for these inherent differences. Any lifestyle prescription must match the individual nature of the person.

1 PHYSIOLOGY

- Unique genetic makeup
- Different epigenetic expression
- Varied endocrine effects
- Variations in disease susceptibility
- Varied hunger, energy, and craving responses
- Individual reactions to metabolic compensation
- Natural proclivities toward energy use and storage

2 PSYCHOLOGY

- Unique personality
- Varied responses to emotional stress
- Different orientations toward rest and work
- Mood-related variations
- Emotional differences
- Natural proclivities toward motivation, drive, productivity, passion, meaning, and purpose
- Variations in resilience and resolve

3 PERSONAL PREFERENCE

- Individual habits
- Likes and dislikes
- Assumptions and expectations
- Life philosophy
- Underlying values
- Perceptions and Perspectives

4 PRACTICAL CIRCUMSTANCES

- Living situation
- Monetary resources
- Intellectual ability
- Physical limitations
- Past traumas
- Educational resources
- Environmental conditions

My solution was to make small modifications that would add up to big results. I made him switch from regular Coke to Diet Coke and from candy bars to protein bars. I suggested he swap out his potato chips for Slim Jims, beef jerky, or boiled eggs. I told him to eat wherever he wanted to but to strip the buns off his burgers and skip fat and carb/sugar combinations such as milkshakes, french fries, and pastries.

Knowing Dale had played football in high school, I gave him a few moves from his training days he could do at rest stops, including one-minute sets of push-ups or air squats at every stop. He thought all this was a little weird but admitted that it sounded doable and said he would give it a try.

I was convinced I would never see him again, but a few months later, Dale was back. He walked into my office, and I honestly did not recognize him. He had lost over twenty-five pounds, was no longer taking his diabetic medication, and was beaming from ear to ear. He excitedly told me how his regular physician was so impressed that he wanted to know what Dale was doing. Dale said, "I told him you put me on the Slim Jim diet, and it has been the easiest diet I have ever done." Although I cringed at the idea of another doctor thinking I put their patient on a diet of Slim Jims and Diet Coke, I also thought it was hilarious. Dale's story is one of the most impactful of my clinical career and illustrates how powerful individualized metabolic tendencies are. You simply can't ignore these four aspects of metabolic individuality and expect to make meaningful progress.

LAW #3: THE LAW OF PSYCHIC ENTROPY

This law states that when you are drained, you have to allow yourself to recharge. In this law, "psychic" means brain and "entropy" means loss of energy—this is more commonly known as "brain drain."

Your brain is like a battery—there are things that drain it and things that charge it, and it's important to be aware of both. A drained brain is a sure sign metabolism is under stress. Unfortunately, many things can contribute to that drain: our never-ending to-do lists, negative people, traffic, chores, TV, diet, exercise, even our own self-awareness and self-editing. The good news is, there are plenty of things that can charge it as well.

This can be anything that quiets that constant mental chatter: massage, music, hot baths, sex, meditation, mindfulness—all of these take us out of our own heads and replenish our energy. Walking in nature is one of the best ways to recharge. By this, I don't mean power walking, which actually can drain your battery as you push yourself to walk fast and burn as many calories as possible. I mean strolling, looking at the trees, taking in your environment, and just enjoying the moment of being outside.

When we experience brain drain, we tend to fall back on shortcut bad habits that put stress on our metabolism: we grab a doughnut, we skip a workout, we make excuses. Habits are the brain's way of creating shortcuts for itself. Those shortcuts are most utilized under times of stress. When we hit "brain drain," we revert back to old habits. We blame these reactions on a lack of willpower. People love to claim they have no willpower when in reality, we all do. And just like the brain, willpower can be drained or charged. I actually prefer to call willpower "skillpower" because building any skill requires practice, and you have to practice building the skill of willpower. You need to understand what actions add more power to your batteries and how to deal with the things that take that power away. Once you do, you are able to create stress Band-Aids that protect you from defaulting to negative habits. We'll dig deeper into the specific ways you can do this in coming chapters, but for now, I just want you to understand that willpower is not something you do or don't have—it's a skill you build over time and continue to strengthen throughout your life. Easy is earned.

This lack of a real end point is true of your entire journey to mastering metabolism. You've only arrived when arrival is no longer the goal. In other words, you're never going to end somewhere; you're always becoming. In fact, the endless attempt to reach some kind of fictional finish line can be one of the biggest drainers of your willpower battery.

If you constantly feel as if you need to get somewhere and are failing because you've not made it yet, you're ultimately beating yourself up over something that doesn't exist.

Comparison is another major energy drainer. You cannot view your own experience through the lens of anyone else's. People often say to me, "Jade, you have it easy because you've been doing this for thirty years. I'll never be like you." I always tell them, "You're right. You'll never be where I am because I have my own metabolic challenges. I have issues with pre-diabetes and cholesterol that you might not have. I have a very specific body type that you probably don't have or want. So no, you are never going to be me. And I'm never going to be you." Everybody has their own journey they're walking, and what it means to feel their best and function at their peak is different for every single person.

THE 4MS

Just as there are four main factors making each of our metabolisms unique, there are four areas we can consciously influence to impact metabolic output: mindset, movement, meals, and metabolics.

Mindset/Mindfulness

Mindset together with mindfulness and movement is the key way to take stress off the system. As mentioned in the explanation of the law of psychic entropy, mindfulness is an ideal way to recharge the battery. Again, this can be walking, particularly in a green setting, listening to music, cuddling with pets, taking a bath, practicing meditation, getting a massage, or stretching. Creative pursuits such as coloring, playing an instrument, and painting have been shown to lower stress in adults. We'll explore mindfulness in more detail in Chapter Nine.

Movement

When I use the term "movement," I am referring to non-exercise activity thermogenesis (remember NEAT from earlier?). I also often use movement and walking as synonyms as walking is by far the biggest contribution to NEAT. As a reminder, movement and exercise are not the same things—exercise is a structured goal to achieve a particular outcome; movement is everything you do to keep your metabolism flexible. Movement is about getting from point A to point B. Exercise is time-bound and

A NOTE ON TV

Notice I did not list watching TV in the list of things that can charge your battery.

That's because different kinds of shows can have varying effects on each person. Comedies, for instance, act like chargers because laughter is a natural way to release stress. Educational things also can be stimulating and lower stress levels. Some things you watch might initially offer a relaxation response but ultimately have a draining effect. For example, if you love scary movies but they leave your heart racing and your pulse pounding, you are anything but relaxed. Furthermore, if every time you sit down to watch your favorite show you also have a bag of chips in hand, that's a problem.

I know a couple who's very busy with work and kids and gets only one night a week to watch TV together. They love true crime shows and tend to spend the evening bingeing on *Dateline*, *Unsolved Mysteries*, and the like. The wife noticed that on those days, the husband munched on snacks all night and she'd end up downing two or three glasses of wine. Their bad habits were totally linked to their viewing habits. It was time to either find something new to watch or figure out a better way to spend their evening together.

The answer is not to stop watching TV altogether. It's about being aware of its impact on you and deciding if what you're watching is worth it.

goal-oriented. Movement is far more important and impactful than exercise. The goal is to move as much as possible and exercise only just enough.

Remember that metabolism is always measuring everything, including the tension on your body. When you're sitting in a chair all day, every day, your metabolism becomes like a weak, frayed rubber band. But when you're walking all day every day and constantly using your muscles—which is what our metabolism is used to from our hunter-gatherer days—your endocrine system instructs the metabolism to become more flexible.

Meals

Meals refers to what you are putting in your mouth.

When it comes to fat loss and body change, meals means much more than nutrition. It's about the quality, quantity, timing, and frequency of the things you eat. What you eat and when you eat play a significant role in how your body responds. For example, if you eat most of your daily allotment of carbohydrates after exercise, you may recover better. If you are more insulin-sensitive first thing in the morning (as most of us are), a doughnut early in the day has less of a negative response than a doughnut at night. Energy-producing macronutrients right before bed might lead to difficulty sleeping. Or maybe eating your biggest meal in the evening results in a good night's sleep and healthier eating habits the next day. All of these things matter to metabolism. The bottom line is, you can read every study and listen to every podcast about what you should and shouldn't eat, but ultimately, your body is going to tell you. We are all different and there is no one-size-fits-all or perfect diet for everyone.

THE 4Ms OF METABOLISM

There are four main categories of metabolic control. Each has distinct mechanisms that allow for metabolic manipulation. Think of these as choices or actions one can take to alter metabolic output. Metabolism is not simply about diet and exercise. Mindfulness and movement have massive impact.

1 MINDFULNESS
Stress reduction

- Conscious acts of recovery, relaxation, and repair
- Sleep, naps, and silent alone time
- Meditation, massage, music
- Relaxing movement (Yin Yoga, Tai chi)
- Creative pursuits, purposeful living
- Time in nature, time with loved ones
- Physical affection, cuddling, sex
- Sauna, spa time, self care
- Reading, laughter, learning
- Anything that lowers stress hormones

2 MOVEMENT
Daily living activities

- Activities of daily living
- Walking, stretching, fidgeting
- Standing rather than sitting
- Walking rather than standing
- Laundry, gardening, housework
- Ancestral humans accumulated 10K to 20K steps daily
- Makes up 15% of metabolic output
- Sensitizes the body to insulin
- Lowers cortisol

3 MEALS
Energy and building blocks

- What we eat
- Food quality and quantity
- Calories and macronutrients
- Vitamins and minerals
- Fiber and water
- Provides energy
- Metabolic building blocks
- You are what you eat

4 METABOLICS
Metabolic stimulation

- Conscious acts of metabolic stimulation
- All forms of exercise
- Supplements
- Herbs and drugs
- Health technologies
- Surgery and other medical interventions

Metabolics

Metabolics is a catchall phrase I use to mean anything that tries to move or stimulate metabolism. This includes exercise as well as things like supplements and drugs. Metabolics can offer major benefits especially when it comes to shaping the body. But they also can easily be overdone. Remember that metabolism is a stress barometer, and metabolics are intended to add only a small, strategic amount of stress so the metabolism can adapt and get stronger. Of the 4Ms, metabolics is the least important for most people and the one that has the most potential for abuse. What many don't realize is that trying to "stimulate," "boost," or "speed" metabolism also usually elevates hunger and cravings. It's not that exercise isn't powerful—it is the one tool we have to shape the body into a more athletic form. It's just that it is more of a shaper than a reducer. What you eat should be your focus for weight loss. Exercise makes sure the weight you lose is mostly fat rather than muscle. That, and its hugely beneficial response on mood and health, is its most valuable contribution.

THE GOLDILOCKS ZONE

Although it's very hard to overdo mindfulness and movement, you absolutely can overdo both metabolics and meals. You also can under-do each of the Ms. You have to aim for the Goldilocks zone in each area: not too much, not too little, but just right. Eating too much or too little is going to cause problems for metabolism, as will exercising too much or too little. This is where most traditional "dieters" go wrong: they do too much metabolics, not enough meals, and completely disregard mindset/mindfulness.

Once you understand each of these four areas, you should be able to rank how well you're doing at each on a scale of one to ten. Maybe you eat very healthily—give yourself a ten. If you are taking advantage of metabolics but not overusing them, that's another ten. If you're not doing anything for mindset/mindfulness, give yourself a zero. Maybe you take only about 5,000 steps per day—that's a five for movement. Now you know where to focus your attention. Instead of trying to double down on diet and exercise, you can aim to incorporate some stress-reducing techniques into your routine and find ways to be moving more throughout each day. Lo and behold, your cravings and hunger become normalized. Your energy is stable, your sleep is on track, and your mood is up. As soon as you know what changes you need to make, you can set yourself on track for always being at your best.

Up until now, you probably thought metabolism was just about diet and exercise. This is a huge mistake and the dieter's main trap. Now you know there are actually four areas you must address, not just two. If I were to prioritize each into a dominance hierarchy for most people, I would say mindfulness and movement come first, as most people are unaware of them and therefore neglect them. Of course, you must always honor your uniqueness, and if you find either meals or metabolics are your biggest block, honor that.

However, if you are someone who scores low in all four areas, it's best to prioritize mindfulness and movement as those are the first steps to taking stress off the system and controlling sleep, hunger, mood, energy, and cravings.

Again, this entire process has to be highly individualized. You must understand the three laws so you can know what your unique metabolism is doing and why. You have to understand the 4Ps and the 4Ms because if you're going to build your own approach to taking your metabolism to the next level, you have to know what areas need your attention and understand that your plan will not mirror anyone else's.

There's an old saying that if all you have is a hammer, everything starts to look like a nail. This hits the nail on the head (pun intended) when it comes to explaining what's going on in the mind of the dieter. To truly master your metabolism, you have to stop being a dieter and start being a detective.

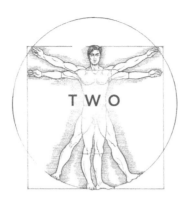

TWO

THE METABOLIC
SCIENTIST

This book is not a diet book, nor is it a medical text. However, a full understanding of metabolism requires that you understand some of the detailed science. This becomes even more critical in understanding the tools, techniques, protocols, and processes I have adopted in my own clinical practice. This chapter will give you a big-picture overview of some of the most important concepts related to metabolism and hormones. But before we get to that, I want to explain several different ways you can understand metabolism.

What is metabolism? Metabolism is the mechanism responsible for seeking, procuring, digesting, assimilating, transporting, and generating energy. Metabolism is your body's energy infrastructure, and just as is the case with any complex system, many factors can impact its function.

SUPPLY AND DEMAND

Oil is the most in-demand fuel source on the planet, and we rely on an entire infrastructure to both get and use it.

Determining where oil might be requires sophisticated equipment. High-tech drills and extraction tubes are used to access and remove the oil. That oil then needs to be transported by boat, train, trucks, and pipelines to areas where it is refined and processed. From there, the oil must once again be shipped to energy centers, gas stations, and homes where it is burned.

The story does not end there. Based on demand, oil consumption can go up or down. These fluctuations tell the entire oil infrastructure to either ramp up its activity or turn it down. This is a classic case of supply and demand.

This is how the metabolism works as well, except multiply the fuel source by five and adjust the complexity by a factor of 1,000. Just as the markets will respond to the supply and demand of oil, the metabolism reacts to the supply of energy and the demands of its environment. In this way, you can think of the metabolism as a computer, a chemistry set, a thermostat, and a stress barometer all in one.

It is constantly measuring the demands placed on it by the outside world (stress barometer), calculating and consuming its energy needs (computer), and then, through a series of complex chemical reactions, producing the energy required (chemistry set) and feeding back to the entire system to make any adjustments (thermostat).

KEY POINTS

- Metabolism is the body's energy management system.
- It works on supply and demand.
- It is complicated and has many interconnected moving parts.
- The metabolism is one big stress-measuring device combined with a sophisticated computer, a chemistry set, and a feedback system like a thermostat.

WHERE IS THE CENTER OF METABOLISM?

The hypothalamus, an area of the brain just above the brain stem, gathers information from the senses and receives hormonal input from the body. It then sends out instructions via nerve signals and hormonal output to control physiology.

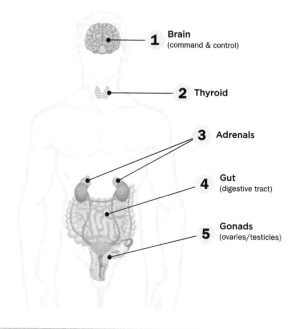

1 Brain
(command & control)

2 Thyroid

3 Adrenals

4 Gut
(digestive tract)

5 Gonads
(ovaries/testicles)

METABOLISM AS SOCIALIZER

To make it even easier to understand metabolism, let's use social interactions. You're human, so you are already an expert in connecting and interacting with other humans. We humans are social creatures above all else, so in this example, "food energy" is synonymous with "social connection."

The metabolism is always seeking balance (what science calls homeostasis). The metabolism seeks just enough food to feel good, look good, function better, and live longer. This means it wants the perfect amount—not too much, not too little, but just right, just like Goldilocks.

This is similar to how you interact socially. You crave a certain amount of interaction. If you have too little social interaction, you will feel lonely, sad, and unsure. If you have too many people around and too many social demands, you can easily become overwhelmed, drained, bitter, unsure, or unproductive.

In order to balance this equation, you will institute all kinds of conscious and unconscious actions. Some days, you might send multiple texts, make some calls, spend hours on social media, and meet friends out for drinks. Other days, you might sit on the couch, screen calls, and avoid social interaction as much as possible.

Left to its own devices, this is how the metabolism works as well. Sometimes it will feel motivated and hungry and desire certain flavors and foods. Other days, it may want to sleep in, eat sparingly, and avoid a lot of activity. This depends on a number of different factors and circumstances during the previous days.

Just like you naturally regulate your social energy and interactions, the metabolism is naturally regulating its energy balance as well. Imagine if you were stuck in solitary confinement for two weeks with no social interaction. Or imagine if you had to spend two weeks straight inside a never-ending, wall-to-wall dance club. Neither of those extremes would feel comfortable. You would likely institute all manner of coping mechanisms as a result.

The same thing happens with the metabolism. Whenever it is confronted with too much or too little, it reacts negatively and does everything it can to get back to balance. Whereas you might get sad and lonely if you were isolated socially, the metabolism gets hungry and loses motivation when it has too little food. You might get agitated and irritable if you are overwhelmed socially. The metabolism suffers disrupted sleep, increased cravings, and unpredictable energy when it is overwhelmed with too much food.

Furthermore, if you watch the same movie every day, hang with the same people, and read the same chapter out of the same book at the same time each and every day, you are not going to feel very mentally stable. In fact, you may go insane. The metabolism is exactly the same. It thrives off change and challenge. It is adaptable by nature and functions best when it is able to freely react to its environment.

Many people think they should have a fast metabolism. What we really want is a flexible and adaptive system. A fast metabolism is one speed, which means it can't change and is too rigid. The healthiest, most functional and lean metabolisms can speed up, slow down, take tight turns, adjust to bumpy terrain, and adjust to the infinite conditions of the road.

KEY POINTS

- The metabolism becomes dysfunctional whenever it is confronted with too much or too little.
- The metabolism seeks balance constantly.
- The metabolism is an adaptive and reactive system.
- The metabolism does not do well under rigid conditions (i.e., the same conditions day in and day out).
- This is why doing the eat less, exercise more approach to dieting ends up causing issues.
- A fast metabolism is not ideal; a flexible metabolism is the ideal.

METABOLISM AS SURVIVAL SOFTWARE

The metabolism is a system dedicated to helping you survive—if you were a computer, the metabolism would be the operating system. Just as a computer gathers information from its keyboard, Wi-Fi, USB drive, mic, and video camera, your metabolism gathers information from its sight, hearing, taste, touch, scent, emotional sense, and digestive function. This information needs to get relayed to the cells deep inside the body so they know how to respond. This happens through nerve impulses and hormones. Think of nerve impulses as text messages or phone calls; think of hormones as little metabolic mail carriers delivering emails and letters.

When the brain sees, hears, or senses something, it writes a message and sends it to the cells of the body, the same way I might send you a quick text asking you to pick up some milk on your way home from work. Or maybe the message is not so urgent, or I want to send it to a lot of different recipients at once. I probably wouldn't call or text for that but rather send out an email to multiple contacts or a letter to everyone involved.

It may seem silly to think of the metabolism in this way, but understanding how it acts as a message system can help you decipher what your metabolism is telling you. If the metabolism is sending the signal of hunger, that is something you can feel. If it is producing high stable and focused energy, it is useful to know what conditions created that. If your sleep is disrupted and fragmented, your mood is off and irritable, and you are having uncontrollable cravings, those are all hints about the state of your metabolism and its current needs.

KEY POINTS

- The metabolism is constantly measuring what is going on in the outside world.
- It uses hormones to tell the inside cells how to respond.
- These hormones are indirectly or directly responsible for producing sensations we can feel.
- SHMEC is our way to measure metabolic stress.
- When SHMEC is in check, we are likely in a flexible stable position.
- When SHMEC is out of check, we are in a rigid, stuck metabolic state.
- When we are flexible, we are thriving.
- When we are rigid, we are rotting.

I call this window into your metabolic computer software SHMEC. SHMEC is an acronym for sleep, hunger, mood, energy, and cravings. When your SHMEC is in check, you can be relatively certain your metabolism is in a state of balance. When your SHMEC is out of check, it is a sign your metabolism is in a state of stress.

ENERGY PRODUCTION AND CELLULAR CASTLES

The metabolism produces energy in cells. You can think of your cells as little remote castles. Like a castle, they are designed to be selective in what they let in and out. They literally have a moat and wall just as a castle does. The cell membrane is a semipermeable barrier that looks for signals from the outside world.

A hormone such as insulin acts like a rider approaching the castle gate and saying, "Hey! Open up! I have some firewood for you." The guards at the gate greet insulin and say, "Thanks so much! Bring it on in." From there, the wood is taken to the fireplaces and forges inside the castle, chopped up, and burned.

Your cell is pretty crafty because it can use lots of different types of firewood. It is like a car that can simultaneously run off diesel, unleaded, jet fuel, and electrical energy as needed. In fact, based on the demands placed on the cell and the fuel available to it, it can mix and match fuel amount and type as needed. The problem comes when you get too much fuel or an excess of the same type of fuel.

Imagine if you were the king of the castle and every time insulin came, he was bringing in massive quantities of a poorly burning fuel. Before you knew it, you would have firewood everywhere disrupting the workings of the castle and spewing black smoke from the chimneys, making life in the castle miserable and unhealthy. The furnaces and forges of your cells are little energy-producing units called mitochondria. They work best when they have enough *but not too much* energy. They also are healthiest when they are given variations in fuel.

You can think of these little mitochondria as sorting houses. When the wood comes in, they clean it, chop it, and get ready to burn it. They have different segments of the factory floor devoted to each type of firewood. If huge quantities of one type of wood are always coming in, all the workers need to be diverted to that task. They get very good at it but become rusty and less efficient at burning other types of fuels. This is what happens when you eat the standard American diet every day, day in and day out. It is also what is likely to happen with any type of dietary regime you do every single day, day after day, year after year, without deviation. In order for your castle to function best, it needs the right amount of fuel and the right type for the right job or season.

KEY POINTS

- The cells of the metabolism respond to hormones and are selective in what they let in and out.
- The cell is like its own little energy-producing city that needs to make energy for itself and the demands of the body.
- The mitochondria in the cells can become overwhelmed and dysfunctional if they are inundated with large amounts of fuel and/or the same types of fuel day in and day out.

METABOLISM AS INDIVIDUAL

The final thing you need to know about the metabolism is that each one is unique because you are unique. Imagine every human body was a different car, each with its own special strengths and different weaknesses. Some would be pure electric vehicles while others would be high-performing sports cars that run off jet fuel. Some are good at off-roading; some do best on the racetrack; others like long drives in the mountains. Some can handle snow and weather wonderfully. Others thrive in extremes of heat and dryness.

This is how your metabolism works as well. You are unique in your physiology, psychology, personal preferences, and practical circumstances. Your metabolism shares a lot of overlap with other humans, but like your fingerprint, it is subtly unique in extremely important ways.

Although it helps to understand what the metabolism is and how it functions, it is most important to discover how your unique metabolism varies and performs. Your metabolic machinery likes to run on a variety of fuels. Some people do best with oats and fruit in the morning. Others thrive with eggs and bacon. Still others function optimally by skipping breakfast altogether.

Up until now, you have likely been operating under the assumption that there is one perfect lifestyle everyone should be following. This is wrong. There is no perfect diet. The perfect diet is created out of a deep understanding of your own metabolic workings, the psychological sensitivities unique to you, and the varied nature of your personal preferences.

The process by which you uncover your metabolic uniqueness and begin to eat, move, think, and live in accordance with that is what I call being metabolic. It is the state of metabolic thriving that only this approach can uncover.

When SHMEC is in check, you are attaining (or maintaining) a lean muscular physique and blood labs and vitals are moving in optimal directions; you have found what works for you. Now, when the metabolism changes, as it always does, you have a process to repeat rather than trying to find another imperfect off-the-shelf one-size-fit-all protocol.

HOW METABOLISM WORKS

Although everyone has a unique metabolism, there are a few things happening in each person that dictate how it functions. The brain, specifically the hypothalamus, is the command-and-control center of the metabolism. Think of the hypothalamus like central command in the military. The hypothalamus is responsible for integrating information from the outside world with the needs and conditions inside the body. It is a hub of activity that receives signals, integrates that information, and sends out its own signals to the rest of the body through nerve impulses and hormonal releasing agents.

Hormones that come from the hypothalamus are often referred to as releasing hormones. Anytime you see RH in an abbreviation, it's a good chance that hormone came from the hypothalamus. They go by names like GnRH (gonadotropin-releasing hormone), TRH (thyrotropin-releasing hormone), and CRH (corticotropin-releasing hormone). These three releasing hormones make up the beginning steps of communication between the brain and the gonads (testes and ovaries), thyroid, and adrenals, respectively.

When the hypothalamus integrates all the signals from outside and inside the body, it sends releasing hormones and nerve signals out to adjust the metabolism. The pituitary receives many of these signals and responds with a host of signaling molecules of its own. The pituitary gland releases stimulating hormones that often have the abbreviation SH, such as FSH/LH (follicle-stimulating hormone and luteinizing hormone), TSH (thyroid-stimulating hormone), and ACTH (adrenocorticotropic hormone). These hormones communicate directly to the gonads, thyroid, and adrenal glands.

The first basic understanding of metabolic science is these three critical hormonal networks. The connection and communication from the hypothalamus to the pituitary and then to the thyroid gland is called the HPT axis (hypothalamic-pituitary-thyroid axis). There is also the HPA axis (hypothalamic-pituitary-adrenal axis) and the HPG axis (hypothalamic-pituitary-gonadal axis).

If the metabolism were a jumbo passenger jet, the hypothalamus would be the pilot in the cockpit, the pituitary would be the copilot, the adrenals and thyroid glands would be the right and left engines, and the gonads would be the tail rudder. The hypothalamus and pituitary work together to "fly" your metabolic airplane. Now, imagine the pilot's instrument panel getting scrambled, flying into a ferocious thunderstorm, encountering extreme turbulence, or a group of hijackers attempting to breach the cockpit. This is analogous to chronic stress, poor dietary inputs, inflammatory insult, and infectious agents. All of these things disrupt the ability of the metabolism to find balance or homeostasis.

If the hypothalamus and pituitary are the president and vice president of the metabolism, then the gut (digestive tract), liver, and immune system are the generals. The gut is a key mover of metabolism and is the five-star general. The liver and immune system are the four-star generals. You can think of all other tissues like muscle, fat tissue, and the rest as the colonels, captains, and lieutenants. All these systems are taking orders from their higher-ups, sending orders down to their platoons (the cells they influence), and reporting back to the brain the conditions on the ground.

How does the metabolism manage all this communication? Hormones!

A QUICK CLARIFICATION FOR THE SERIOUS SCIENCE NERDS

The term "hormone" in biochemistry classically refers to a chemical released by a gland or cell in one part of the body that then travels through the blood and binds to cell receptors in other parts of the body. The most popular of these hormones are the steroid hormones that include sex steroids (estrogen, progesterone, testosterone), stress steroids (like cortisol), and regulatory hormones (like aldosterone). However, the definition of hormone has been expanded to include other signaling molecules that don't function exactly this same way. To make matters simple, the term "hormone" I am using here is meant to denote all signaling molecules in the body.

The metabolism communicates through signaling molecules. When the immune system needs to signal certain immune cells to an area of injury or infection, it uses cytokines. When the fat cell needs to communicate to the brain, it releases adipokines. When the muscle sends signals about demands placed upon it, it uses myokines. The brain uses neurotransmitters. The gut uses incretins. And so on. All of these compounds have hormone-like action because they are released from one area and communicate to other areas locally or at distant body sites. The brain, gut, and immune system are a few of the biggest hotbeds of this metabolic communication.

You can think of these signaling molecules as phone calls, text messages, emails, DMs, and handwritten letters. The hormonal system is the metabolism's communication network.

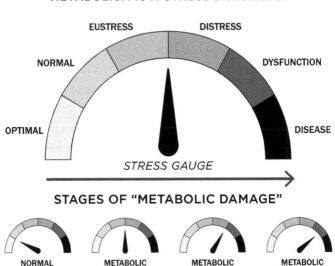

METABOLISM IS A STRESS BAROMETER

EUSTRESS   DISTRESS

NORMAL   DYSFUNCTION

OPTIMAL   DISEASE

STRESS GAUGE

STAGES OF "METABOLIC DAMAGE"

NORMAL HOMEOSTASIS   METABOLIC COMPENSATION   METABOLIC RESISTANCE   METABOLIC DYSFUNCTION

The major role of metabolism as a whole is as one big sensing and responding apparatus. What is it sensing? Stress! How does it respond? In a way that restores balance or homeostasis. If the metabolism is one big stress barometer, its job is to make sure the pressure is not too much, not too little, but just right. This means the communication channels must remain clear and unobstructed. That is incredibly difficult when you are dealing with extreme or chronic stress.

WHAT IS THE BEST ANALOGY FOR METABOLISM?

The metabolism gathers information from the environment (light, food, temperature, threats, etc.) and integrates that with input from the cells (energy needs, cellular signals, etc.) and then plots an appropriate course of action by adapting, reacting, and adjusting its responses to meet the needs of the body. It is a measuring and responding apparatus. What's it measuring and responding to? Stress!

METABOLISM IS:

- Creative
- Responsible
- Adaptive
- Unpredictable
- Multiple means of feedback (i.e., hunger, energy, cravings)
- Changeable
- Unconscious
- Inconsistent

Calculator	Chemistry Set	Speedometer	Thermostat*
✕ Predictable	✓ Predictable	✕ Predictable	✓ Predictable
✕ Repeatable	✕ Repeatable	✕ Repeatable	✓ Repeatable
✕ Reliable	✕ Reliable	✓ Reliable	✓ Reliable
✕ Consistent	✕ Consistent	✕ Consistent	✕ Consistent
✓ Feedback	✓ Feedback	✓ Feedback	✓ Feedback

* Human metabolism is one of the most complex systems known to man. If we are going to try to apply a simple analogy to the metabolism, which we really shouldn't, the thermostat analogy is probably the closest fit.

THREE TIERS OF METABOLISM

To make it as simple as possible, think of metabolism as consisting of three tiers or compartments. Compartment one is the brain level. It consists of nerve impulses and the hypothalamic-pituitary axis (the HPT, HPA, and HPG). Compartment two is the tissue level (muscle, fat, skeleton, gut, liver, kidney, immune, etc.). Compartment three is the individual cells including the end unit of energy production called the mitochondria. These are the small organelles in every cell responsible for making the energy your metabolism consumes to stay alive and thrive.

While the brain is taking in all the information from the outside world, it has to integrate that information with the signaling it receives from the tissues and cells. From there, it begins instituting its plan. Of course, there is all kinds of information being communicated, but to keep things simple, let's focus on the most important: the gap between the amount of energy the metabolism is burning and the amount it has available. I call this the calorie gap. There are many different types of stress the metabolism responds to, but perhaps the biggest stress is the discrepancy between the resources the metabolism needs to survive and how many of those resources it has. If there is one single mission of the metabolism, it is to stay alive long enough to reproduce. Historically speaking, the major impediments to that goal were starvation, infection, and injury. Here, we are focusing on starvation. Anytime the body perceives a lack of energy resources, especially when it comes in the context of increased metabolic demand, it jumps into action.

THE GAP BETWEEN CALORIE INTAKE AND CALORIE OUTPUT IS A MAJOR METABOLIC STRESSOR

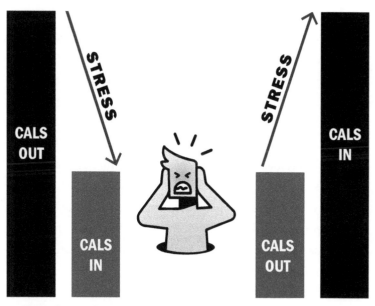

Eating less and exercising more and eating more and exercising less widen the calorie gap and may register as a stress to the metabolism.

The first thing the body does is increase food-seeking behavior. Hormones like ghrelin, cortisol, and others signal back to the brain, reducing motivational centers, increasing reward-seeking behavior, and elevating hunger in general—most specifically, cravings for calorie-rich foods.

Before food even enters the mouth, the process of digestion, absorption, and assimilation begins. When you see a food, the brain has memory of it and expectations for it. Looking at a steak and smelling it cooking on a fire kick off the memory of certain textures and flavors. Those textures and flavors carry memories of certain nutrients (in this case, amino acids), and the metabolism begins prepping the body with increased salivation, hydrochloric acid, and pepsin secretion in the stomach. Once you begin chewing the food, the brain adds to the information it has. It says, "Not only did that look and smell like steak, but it also now chews and tastes like steak." That amplifies the digestive process.

When you swallow that steak, the digestive secretions in the stomach go to work. As the stomach expands, stretch receptors in the stomach signal the brain about how much food it should expect. The stomach also releases certain hormones that tell the brain to slow eating and feel full. As the food passes from the stomach to the intestine, pancreatic enzymes and bile enter the mix. Surprisingly, the body continues to "taste" your food long after it has left your mouth. L and K cells lining the small intestines sample/feel/taste the digestive contents and start firing off incretin hormones like GIP and GLP. These hormones are powerful movers of metabolism that communicate to the pancreas about insulin need and shut down hunger in the brain. As the food continues moving through the small intestines, other hunger hormones further down like PYY start sending "stop eating" signals to the brain.

As the digested contents start moving from the gut to the bloodstream, the signals about what and how much was eaten continue to be released. The first place the digested material goes is the liver. And again, the liver sends its own messages while also continuing to receive instructions from the brain and other tissues about what is needed. From there, the liver starts adjusting energy needs. It moves from producing glucose (gluconeogenesis) to consuming and storing it (glycogen synthesis). Other tissues burn the energy they can immediately use and begin storing any leftovers. If the intake exceeds what the body can currently use, the extra is stored as glycogen (the body's version of potato starch), muscle (the metabolism's amino acid pantry), and fat (the largest storage depot). These tissues all then send feedback to the other tissues explaining their current metabolic state and needs.

As the meal travels into the large intestines, bacteria begin to digest the leftovers. Depending on the diversity and type of bacteria you have, more signaling molecules are released. The bacteria living in the human gut are more numerous than cells in the human body. These bacteria have profound impact on metabolic function as well as producing compounds that can influence mood, hunger, cravings, and the rest. They are also a source of extra nutrition-synthesizing compounds like butyrate that act as fuel for the body, especially the cells lining the digestive tract. The bacteria inhabiting your gut are known as your microbiome, and many scientists now regard the microbiome as perhaps the largest and most important organ in the human body, even though it is technically outside of the body and not made up of human cells at all. Although this area of research is extremely interesting and provides a huge reservoir of untapped metabolic understanding, we are still in our infancy in terms of understanding how to measure or manipulate it. Your microbiome is somewhat like a fingerprint and may hold the key to metabolic manipulations that may keep you lean, fit, and optimally healthy. Unfortunately, the science is too new to have any definitive directions regarding the microbiome other than the theory that a healthy, lean, fiber-based diet may be best for helping it function optimally.

Once your food reaches the cell, it moves into the mitochondria. You can think of your mitochondria as car engines that can simultaneously burn jet fuel (carbs) and diesel fuel (fat) as well as flex fuel (protein). They can also burn a few other sources of energy such as alcohol and ketones. They do this by breaking most of these fuels down into one universal fuel called acetyl-CoA, especially carbs, fats, and alcohol.

Acetyl-CoA then gets broken down into smaller and smaller molecules in a cellular process resembling a waterwheel. As acetyl-CoA is broken down, energy is released. Think of this as a spinning wheel generating sparks. These "sparks" or energy packets get picked up by little intracellular taxis (NAD and FADH). The "sparks" are then shuttled into the inner mitochondria where the energy is passed around like a hot potato from one energy-producing protein to another. Along the way, an energy gradient builds up across the mitochondrial membrane, which becomes the battery power that produces an energy packet called ATP. That ATP is then used to power the entire cellular city.

This process can either be clean and efficient or dirty and damaging. If you consume a pizza and beer dinner followed by a giant cheesecake, the mitochondrial shuttles and delicate machinery can become overwhelmed, kicking off excess free radicals and pushing the cells' antioxidant systems to the brink. You can think of free radicals like flaming meteors that go zipping around the cells tearing functional proteins apart. You can think of antioxidants as giant catcher's mitts that intercept these free radicals and neutralize them before they can do damage.

All of this then gets fed back into the metabolic system by the cells themselves. At this point, the chain of metabolic command is reversed with the foot soldiers (mitochondria) reporting to the platoon sergeants (cells), which then send their signals out to the lieutenants, colonels, and captains (body tissues) and then up to the generals (gut) and the commander in chief, the brain (hypothalamus). From there, once again the hypothalamus integrates the situation in the body with the demands of the outside world, measuring the stress at both ends and plotting a course to restore balance once more.

FOUR STEPS OF FAT BURNING

To lose or gain fat, there must be a discrepancy between the energy coming into the body and the energy the body is using—either a calorie deficit or calorie excess. When too much energy is coming in and not enough is being burned, this is known as a hypercaloric state. When too little energy is coming in compared to what's being burned, this is called a hypocaloric state. Both hypocaloric and hypercaloric states represent a calorie gap to the metabolism. When energy in and out are equal, this is known as an isocaloric state.

For fat to be burned, you must achieve a hypocaloric state. However, if the calorie gap gets too wide for too long, this can register as stress to the metabolism. More specifically, it is a signal of starvation. And starvation is not necessarily the signal you want the metabolism to be responding to as that signal involves hormonal alarm bells characterized by increased cortisol, reduced thyroid activity, and increased expression of ghrelin with decreased leptin signaling. Translation? Reductions in metabolic rate, elevations in hunger and cravings, drops in energy, and negative effects on mood and sleep, among others.

To avoid this, you want to work with the body by either exposing it to extreme but very short-lived calorie deficits or, alternatively, very gentle and prolonged calorie deficits.

In this case, the hormonal signals from the brain cause the four-step process of fat burning. First, fat releases from a fat cell (lipolysis). Second, fat travels through the blood stream to the tissue that needs energy. Third, fat enters into the cell. And finally, fourth, fat burns in the mitochondria (i.e., lipid oxidation). It is important to realize that just because fat is released from a cell (lipolysis) does not mean it will ultimately be burned in the cell (lipid oxidation). In fact, it can easily be restored. This is a very common misunderstanding. Virtually the entire weight loss industry speaks as if lipolysis and lipid oxidation are the same thing. Understanding that they are different helps you realize why some things work while others don't.

This is why hormonal effects are so important. Insulin resistance, among other metabolic imbalances, is characterized by increased blood sugar and blood fats (i.e., triglycerides). Lipolysis may be occurring, but lipid oxidation is compromised—a situation where fat is being released but cannot be adequately burned.

The science of metabolism is a closely orchestrated and extremely complex and refined process. We know only a tiny fraction of the signaling molecules involved and therefore are unable to measure or manipulate metabolism in the ways we often think we can. This is why understanding the ultimate functions and aims of metabolism is critical. Hormones directly or indirectly impact sensations like sleep, hunger, mood, energy, cravings, digestion, mental focus, exercise performance, menses, libido, erections, and every conceivable sign or symptom including joint pain, headaches, and all the rest. This simple understanding, along with knowing whether you are losing weight or gaining weight, tells us the two things most critical to attaining fat loss: caloric load and hormonal balance.

4 STAGES OF FAT BURNING

Fat breakdown
and release
(lipolysis)

Restored?

Triglyceride
travels through
blood stream

Fat enters cell

Energy
CO_2
H_2O_2

Fat is burned
inside cell
(lipid oxidation)

The biofeedback sensations mentioned above tell about hormonal balance. Whether we are losing fat or not tells us whether we have achieved a calorie deficit or not. In fact, weight loss is the only way to know for sure we are in a calorie deficit. This is why discussions of metabolic mechanisms are less useful than you might have initially thought and why understanding the way your metabolism functions and the language it speaks is more important.

A HORMONE IN ACTION

To illustrate how all this works, let's use thyroid hormone as a model. I am using thyroid hormone because it is one of the more complex hormones and illustrates the metabolic cascade, the hormonal feedback system, and cellular handling of hormones all at the same time. It is also one of the most important hormones for those interested in metabolic weight loss to understand.

It starts with the hypothalamus and pituitary glands both receiving information about how much thyroid hormone is in circulation. If we go back to the pilot and copilot example, you can think of the pituitary as reading the instrument display that indicates T4 and T3 levels (T4 thyroxine and T3 triiodothyronine are the major thyroid hormones). The hypothalamus is also sensing these levels but integrating other information like how much fat is stored on the body (signaled by a hormone called leptin) as well as metabolic demands like stress, light, temperature, and other parameters. Together, the pilot (hypothalamus) and copilot (pituitary) plot a course for thyroid output.

The hypothalamus releases TRH (thyrotropin-releasing hormone—some people call this thyroid-releasing hormone for short). The pituitary senses TRH. It also measures and senses its own levels of thyroid hormone. It then integrates the signals from the hypothalamus along with its own thyroid levels and releases TSH. In this way, you can think of the hypothalamus as the stress barometer and the pituitary as the thermostat.

TSH then travels to the thyroid gland where it signals the thyroid gland to start making and releasing more thyroid hormone. Thyroid hormones are basically a combination of the amino acid tyrosine with iodine molecules. T4, or thyroxine, is essentially tyrosine combined with four iodine molecules. T3, or triiodo-thyronine, is thyroxine with one less iodine molecule. Both hor-mones are made in the follicular cells of the thyroid gland using a host of proteins and cofactors. Thyroglobulin and thyroid perox-idase are two of those proteins. This process also requires iodine, tyrosine, and other nutrients.

From there, the thyroid gland releases mainly T4 and only small amounts of T3. This is where things get interesting and com-plicated. T4 is largely regarded as a hormonal reservoir because it is not the primary thyroid hormone that drives action inside the cell. T3 is the primary thyroid hormone. T3, the active hormone, is created from T4 by removing an iodine molecule. This is accom-plished by deiodinases residing in different tissues. There are three major types—D1, D2, and D3. Much of thyroid conversion from T4 to T3 happens in the liver, kidney, and gut. This is accom-plished by D1. The active thyroid hormone generated by D1 seems to be exported to the plasma for use around the body.

However, there is also T3 generated inside tissues that seems to be for local use by the cell. This T3 is generated from T4 by D2. This is an important and underappreciated aspect of thyroid phys-iology. It used to be thought that all active thyroid hormone was converted from T4 to T3 in the liver and kidneys, then exported to the blood where it was delivered to other cells. Certainly, some of that is occurring, but many cells are controlling their own thyroid levels locally. This means one can have low thyroid in the blood and perhaps adequate thyroid in the tissues, or more likely the opposite—normal thyroid in the blood and hypothyroid at the level of certain cells and tissues.

D3 is mostly responsible for turning T4 into inactive T3 (known as reverse T3) and T3 into inactive T2 (D1 has some of these actions as well). The major point to understand is the exquisite and redundant mechanisms needed to activate and deactivate thyroid hormones in the blood and in the tissues.

Another part of this story has to do with the fact that thyroid hormones do not just pass into cells passively but rather must use active transporters. These transporters have different affinities and efficiencies depending on the tissue. For example, the pituitary gland seems to have transporters for thyroid intake that are more efficient than cells elsewhere in the body. This means the pituitary could be picking up adequate thyroid signals (from the hypothalamus and its own internal thyroid levels), while other tissues in the body are registering low thyroid levels. This is called cellular or tissue-specific hypothyroid, and its ramifications are profound. Normal or abnormal thyroid levels cannot be perfectly inferred by TSH and serum thyroid hormones.

There are some ways to determine whether you are dealing with primary hypothyroid (a problem in the thyroid gland itself), secondary hypothyroid (a problem at the level of the feedback and responding apparatus in the brain, i.e., hypothalamus and pituitary), or hypothyroid as a result of decreased thyroid action at the tissues (cellular- or tissue-level hypothyroid).

The pituitary gland, which is responsible for generating the TSH signal, is seen as more sensitive to T4 compared to other tissues. This is because the thyroid hormone transporters in the pituitary gland are different and slightly more efficient (do not require energy) compared to those in other tissues (TR-b2 in pituitary versus TR-b1 and TR-a1 in other tissues). It is also because the pituitary has more D2 and less D1 and D3. This means it can get more T4 in and produce more T3 without conversion to inactivated forms. All this means the pituitary can be sensing normal T4 levels and producing normal T3 levels while other tissues are not.

A cellular danger response at the level of cells may be a trigger for cellular hypothyroid. When a cell is "under stress," it often reduces metabolic output and diverts resources to self-preservation and conservation as opposed to optimal metabolic output. What could cause a cellular stress response? Inflammation, infection, toxicity, reduced energy from diets, high stress hormones, reduced energy from overexercising, and more. This then causes the cell to decrease its uptake of T4 and T3, although the transporters for entry into the cells for T3 are more efficient than those for T4. This causes an increased conversion of thyroid hormones into RT3 and T2 both in the cell and in the blood.

What all this means is that blood tests for thyroid function would begin showing a rising T4 and RT3 at a faster rate compared to T3. This makes the free T3 to reverse T3 level a great surrogate marker for those experiencing low thyroid symptoms but with normal TSH and free T4 and free T3.

Here is a direct excerpt from a research review on the physiology:

Cellular thyroid levels do not correlate with serum levels if uptake into the cells is hindered. This occurs with chronic stress, depression, chronic dieting, diabetes, insulin resistance (obesity) or high cholesterol levels. Thus, with such conditions, TSH, T4 and T3 levels are not accurate measures of intracellular thyroid levels and cannot be used as reliable markers to determine the need for thyroid hormone supplementation.

T4 uptake (utilization) drops much faster than T3 utilization as severity increases, making T4 replacement inappropriate for such conditions. Reverse T3 mirrors T4 uptake so high or high-normal reverse T3 is a marker for reduced uptake of T4 into the cell (and to a lesser extent T3) showing that there is a reduced overall tissue thyroid level requiring T3 supplementation (not T4). Utilizing the free T3/reverse T3 ratio does not suffer from the inaccuracies of standard tests and most closely correlates with cellular thyroid levels...Among patients with this type of thyroid hormone transport dysfunction (resulting in intracellular hypothyroidism) assessing the free T3/reverse T3 ratio can aid in a proper diagnosis, with a free T3/reverse T3 ratio of less than 0.2 being a marker for tissue hypothyroidism (when the free T3 is expressed in pg/mL (2.3–4.2 pg/mL) and the reverse T3 is expressed in ng/dL (8–25 ng/dL).[7]

Another useful lab measure for tissue-level hypothyroidism is the steroid hormone binding globulin (SHBG). SHBG is a binding protein for androgens (testosterone) and estrogen. It is produced in the liver and released from the liver in response to thyroid hormone and estrogen. This gives us a window into thyroid action. If the thyroid levels are adequate, we should expect an SHBG to not be low but instead be normal or high-normal. Low SHBG levels (less than 70 nmol/L in women and 25 nmol/L in men) are another hint that thyroid adequacy in the cells is compromised.

Researchers also suspect that tissue-level hypothyroid is having a critical impact on weight regain after fat loss due to changes in type 1 (D1) deiodinase in the liver and type 3 (D3) deiodinase in the muscle. After weight loss, D3 activity in the muscle ramps up activity, causing T4 to convert to reverse T3 and T3 to be made into T2. This has a net effect of decreasing active thyroid and inducing tissue-level hypothyroid at the level of the muscle.[8]

One final indicator of subclinical or tissue-level hypothyroid may be homocysteine. Elevated homocysteine levels have been correlated with subclinical hypothyroid as well.[9]

Hashimoto's thyroid is a final case to consider in hypothyroid. This is an autoimmune condition where it is believed the immune system is attacking and destroying thyroid tissue. It is diagnosed when hypothyroid symptoms are confirmed with low TSH and high antibodies against the TPO enzyme and/or thyroglobulin protein. Conventional treatment for Hashimoto's hypothyroid is exactly the same as for regular hypothyroid and therefore the distinction is less important. However, I, and other functional medicine doctors like me, have treated Hashimoto's through addressing the gut and its relationship with the immune system. Nutraceuticals also have a potent role to play here. One study on myoinositol (600 mg) and selenium (83 ug) restored the antibodies normally present in Hashimoto's to normal thyroid status.[10] Selenium alone at 200 mcg daily for twelve months and photobiomodulation (i.e., red-light therapy, at 850 NM applied to the thyroid twice daily for three days) also have been shown to be effective. In fact, the two latter treatments have been shown to reduce or eliminate antibodies against thyroid and reduce or eliminate the need for medication in a sizable portion of study participants.[11]

Thyroid Hormone and Fat Loss

Part of the reason I went through all the details of thyroid hormone physiology is because it illustrates a huge degree of complexity as it relates to hormonal influences on metabolism. When it comes to hormones, especially major metabolic regulators like thyroid hormone, we need to appreciate the feedback and feedforward mechanisms (i.e., the HPT axis). We need to appreciate thyroid physiology and the precursors required to make hormone in the gland. We then need to consider transport and regulation in the blood as well as uptake by the tissues and binding to the receptors (i.e., transporters and receptors) and then cellular-level controls of these hormones in the cell (deiodinase activity in the case of thyroid hormone).

Although every hormone is different, at least a few or all of these considerations are at play. This is why single hormones and their mechanisms are woefully inadequate to explain metabolism. Single hormones are complex as illustrated above for the thyroid gland. Hormones don't work in isolation. For example, cortisol, estrogen, testosterone, leptin, and others are just a few hormones that impact thyroid hormone and are impacted by thyroid hormone. This is important because hormones are like people and behave differently depending on whom they are socializing with. Furthermore, we cannot possibly know all the signaling molecules in the body and all the myriad ways those hormones are interacting, communicating, and being regulated.

The take home here is to understand the dramatic role hormones are playing but also to understand that "hormonal metabolic balance" is often best assessed through the way you look, feel, and perform. If you feel vital, have optimal body composition, and vitals and blood labs are moving in optimal directions, then you can be sure you are achieving the two things required for sustained fat loss: hormonal balance and enough but not too much energy intake.

CRASH COURSE IN OTHER METABOLIC HORMONES

So as not to turn this book into a complete biochemistry text, the rest of this hormonal discussion will touch on important metabolic hormones in only a general way. This is designed to give you a taste of hormonal interactions and importance without overwhelming you but also to teach you enough not to become a mechanism chaser (i.e., narrow-mindedly focusing on one hormone and one mechanism of that hormone, such as insulin and its fat-storing action).

Insulin

Insulin is thought to be a powerful fat-storing hormone. In fact, the carbohydrate-insulin hypothesis has dominated much of the talk in weight loss over the last twenty years. In case you are unfamiliar with this hypothesis, its central premise goes like this: it's carbohydrates, *not* calories, that drive fat accumulation and weight gain. This is because insulin has multiple mechanisms that hinder fat burning in muscle and reduce fat release from fat tissue. Because insulin is stimulated most by carbohydrates, high carbohydrate diets lead to high insulin levels, insulin resistance, and fat accumulation. In short, this hypothesis says it's the type of food—carbohydrates—that matters most, not the amount of food.

This hypothesis has led many weight loss practitioners to advise lowering insulin levels as much as possible. This has also spawned many different dietary approaches including paleo, keto, carnivore, fasting, and others. In fact, back in 2010 when I wrote my first book on metabolism (*The Metabolic Effect Diet*), I leaned heavily on the carbohydrate-insulin hypothesis. Today, the most serious students of metabolism regard the hypothesis thoroughly vetted and decidedly wrong. Study after study simply has not proven the primacy of insulin but rather continues to point to calories as the most important thing in fat loss.

It's impossible to separate insulin from calories or quality and quantity of food. They are inextricably linked, and you cannot have one without the other. Insulin and calories are basically the same thing. Calorie type and amount impact insulin, and insulin impacts calories. Insulin plays a role like all hormones do. And yes, insulin is a central figure in metabolism. But understanding insulin goes way beyond just lowering it and is impossible without looking at insulin and calories in context.

Like most hormones, balancing insulin is about having enough but not too much. It is about the lifestyle context of the individual. It is about both quantity and quality of food, as well as the right balance of stress, recovery, rest, and exercise. With hormones, it's all about the Goldilocks effect—not too much, not too little, but just right. That's true of insulin as well.

Balancing insulin means understanding insulin sensitivity and insulin resistance. Hormonal sensitivity means that receptors designed to interact with hormones are in adequate numbers and responding normally. Hormones are essentially nothing more than cellular messengers. If a messenger comes to your house, they will ring the doorbell to let you know they have arrived. That triggers you to get up off the couch and let the messenger in. Depending on what that messenger tells you, you will begin to take certain actions. Perhaps they tell you a tornado is heading your way. In that case, you board up the house, bring the dog inside, and usher all the kids into the basement. Your ability to hear the doorbell and go and talk to the messenger, receive their message, and take the appropriate actions is analogous to hormone sensitivity.

But what if things in the house are dysfunctional? Maybe you have a teenager who has his stereo cranked up. And maybe at the same time your husband is in the backyard with a chainsaw cutting up a fallen tree. Maybe you have the TV on while you're preparing dinner and you're talking to your mother who is concerned about the health of your father. With all that other stuff going on, you would be lucky to hear the doorbell, and even if you did, you may not hear or completely understand what the messenger at the door is trying to tell you. That's analogous to hormone resistance.

When a tissue becomes resistant to a hormone, it means the signal is either not heard or not understood. If that happens, the metabolism can't carry on its normal function and things start to become disturbed. In the case of insulin, being insulin-resistant means blood sugar is not cleared from the body quickly. Rather than reaching the cells, it stays in circulation. This causes direct damage and may also trigger other issues like hunger, cravings, and disrupted energy. Although the term "insulin resistance" is familiar to most, it is almost always misunderstood. To help you understand it better, let's start with looking at insulin from a historical point of view.

Insulin Resistance throughout History

Interestingly, insulin resistance does not merely occur as a result of high insulin levels. Contrary to popular thought, insulin resistance can exist in the presence of low insulin levels as well as high insulin levels.[12] So what exactly is insulin resistance doing? Does it have a purpose? How could both an overfed and starvation state induce it? If we look at insulin through the lens of how the metabolism evolved, we expect to find a survival benefit of insulin resistance. And indeed, we do. Insulin resistance is related to survival, especially in free-living mammals that are preparing for hibernation. Animals like bears, squirrels, and other mammals show insulin resistance similar to humans, beginning in the summer months and progressing as they near hibernation.

Insulin resistance may begin naturally in the summer months when food is plentiful and insulin levels begin to rise. During this time of the year, the days are long, and animals are very active, so the higher calories and insulin levels promote both fat gain and the maintenance of muscle mass. As late summer drifts into fall, insulin and calorie levels rise further as more food, especially starchy food, becomes available in the form of fruits, tubers, and squashes. These high-calorie, starch-loaded foods raise insulin further. Days also become shorter and colder in the fall, reducing activity levels. Since the muscle mass of an individual determines 40 percent of their insulin sensitivity and 70–90 percent of blood glucose clearance, this lack of movement is a big issue. Walking increases glucose receptors on the surface of muscle cells. This is exactly what insulin signals cells to do. Because walking can help muscle clear glucose from the blood without insulin, walking can decrease the need for insulin, decrease its levels, and reverse insulin resistance.

Decreased movement as well as a rich supply of high-carbohydrate plant foods in the fall would greatly impact insulin sensitivity. Sustained high insulin levels, or hyperinsulinemia, is what causes the insulin-resistant state. The combination of hyperin-sulinemia, high calorie loads, and progressing insulin resistance is the perfect scenario for fat storing, ensuring all calories consumed would be preferentially stored rather than burned immediately for fuel. This may seem like a bad thing, but for any wild animal facing down an approaching winter, it would be a key survival advantage.

The rich supply of food present in the summer and fall would come to an abrupt halt in winter. In prehistoric days, winter was a time of few food resources. The drastic reduction in calories would act as a primer for human physiology. Maintaining insulin resistance through the winter could serve as protection. Insulin's action on the liver is to blunt sugar production (gluconeogenesis), but during times of starvation and fasting, this is exactly what you need. By maintaining insulin resistance at the level of the liver and fat tissue, the body would be able to use stored fat and muscle protein to make sugar.

Interestingly, low insulin levels and a persistence of insulin resistance characterize diseases of starvation like anorexia. Research has shown that an abrupt switch to a very low-calorie or low-carb diet can aggravate insulin resistance.[13] This seems to lend credibility to the idea that insulin resistance is a physiological state that evolved as a survival mechanism. However, if the fluctuation in seasonal availability of food is a predictor of insulin levels and sensitivity, then we might also expect to see a relationship between insulin and light, sleep, and activity. It is already a well-established fact that exercise and movement are highly correlated with insulin sensitivity, but the associations with light and sleep are less well known.

Circadian rhythm, the natural physiological attunement to the dark and light cycles, also impacts insulin. Seasonal temperature varies as does the degree of light exposure throughout the year. In the natural world, the summer months have long days and short nights, limiting available hours of sleep. Winter presents the opposite—long nights and short days.

A degree of insulin resistance in both seasons would make sense for survival. In the late summer and early fall, a hyper-insulinemic and an insulin-resistant state would be a perfect adaptation toward storing fat for the coming winter. In the winter, a hypo-insulinemic state along with insulin resistance would ensure all resources available were mobilized to supply the body with energy to survive winter, a period of less food availability.

Seasonal fluctuations in daylight intensity and day length would impact not only what foods are available but movement patterns as well, both of which strongly impact insulin sensitivity. Winter means less movement and very little food. Summer means lots of movement and lots of food. Fall, with lots of food and declining movement, would be the perfect scenario for enhanced fat storing. Likewise, spring, with its increasing food supply and rising movement patterns, would have the opposite effect.

Studies show that seasons influence insulin resistance.[14] Weight gain in preparation for winter by animals parallels physiological changes seen in diabetes in humans. In animals, this situation is acute and protective, but in humans, it becomes chronic and degenerative because the modern-day environment resembles a perpetual late summer and autumn: decreased movement and abundant food.[15] This leads to insulin resistance on a chronic continuous basis and eventually to obesity and type 2 diabetes.

The approach of almost all popular weight loss programs is to address obesity and insulin resistance by lowering calories. This does mimic a winter environment and would be a great course of action IF it could be sustained for several months, but most people are unable to continue eating less for more than a few days or weeks. Instead, they revert quickly back to eating more and moving less.

Insulin Resistance in Different Tissues

Tissue-specific insulin resistance is a more accurate description of what's really going on with insulin.[16] The liver, muscle, fat tissue, brain, and pancreas can all develop dysfunction in insulin signaling. Which tissue is resistant to insulin is impacted by both genetic and lifestyle factors. The degree of systemic insulin resistance and diabetes is determined by which tissues lose insulin sensitivity.

Muscle may be the first tissue that develops insulin resistance due to lack of movement. This would lend credibility to the evolutionary discussion and the development of increased fat depots for survival in winter. As days shorten and temperatures drop, movement would also decrease, and muscle function would suffer. After all, muscle is responsible for 70–90 percent of post-meal glucose disposal. Without movement, a large glucose burden is shifted to adipose tissue and liver.

The liver seems to develop the problem through several mechanisms including local defects in lipoprotein lipase (LPL) function (visceral adipose tissue and/or compromised glycogen storage in the muscles). Adipose tissue sensitivity is tricky, with visceral fat behaving differently than subcutaneous adipose tissue. One thing is certain: as adipose tissue increases in size, especially belly fat, the insulin resistance syndrome is dramatically enhanced through fat cell signaling molecules like TNF-alpha and other adipokines (i.e., signaling molecules released by fat). As fat tissue grows in response to increased food intake or decreased movement, hormones derived from fat cells, like leptin, resistin, and adiponectin, will have direct impacts on other tissues' abilities to properly interact with insulin. Liver and muscle tissues are keenly sensitive to these fat cell-derived signaling molecules.

Some research suggests visceral adiposity secretes more resistin (decreases insulin sensitivity), while subcutaneous fat expresses more adiponectin (enhances insulin sensitivity).[17] This may allow the subcutaneous fat to remain more receptive to insulin as the visceral fat remains more resistant. This also highlights how different fat depots differentially impact systemic resistance to insulin.

Ironically, some studies on insulin resistance in peripheral fat show there is actually a protection from obesity when peripheral fat becomes resistant to insulin.[18] From a fat-storing point of view, resistance to insulin at the level of fat would result in less fat storage and more fat release. This makes sense as the role of insulin in fat is to decrease lipolysis (fat breakdown) in favor of lipogenesis (fat storage).

Research is unclear as to which tissues are affected first and why, but it appears resistance at the level of the muscle and fat is less detrimental than resistance at the level of the liver.[19] When the liver loses its ability to respond to insulin, all the systemic effects like low HDL, high triglycerides, and fasting hyperglycemia begin to occur. It is likely these tissue-specific differences are based to some degree on genetics but obviously are impacted by the environment as well. The important thing would be to deal with the tissue that is most in need to halt the chain of metabolic dysfunction.

Knowing where the primary site of insulin resistance has developed allows one to address that tissue. Researchers have used glucose tolerance tests paired with insulin measures to pinpoint where insulin resistance is most centered.[20] They have used this technique as a way of distinguishing muscle resistance from liver resistance. A fast and large rise of blood sugar in a glucose tolerance test, followed by a sharp decline (i.e., sharp peaks in the blood glucose curve) may indicate insulin resistance primarily in the liver. This is because insulin's normal action on the liver is to stop the production of new sugar (gluconeogenesis) and halt the breakdown of stored sugar (glycogenolysis). If the liver is resistant to insulin, the opposite would occur. Gluconeogenesis and glycogen breakdown would continue. This may cause a high fasting blood sugar and much larger glucose spikes in response to a meal. A blood sugar increase that stayed elevated for long periods after eating (i.e., plateaus) may point to insulin resistance in muscle tissue. Muscle is the primary mover of glucose out of the blood due to its rich supply of glucose transporters. Of course, many people may exhibit a combination of the two (i.e., mountains), pointing toward insulin resistance in both areas. And of course, the normal response would be a valley with lower hills (glucose stays low and only jumps up slightly, then falls back to normal). These trends are easy to see when using a continuous glucose monitor (I will discuss this tool in greater detail later).

Given this understanding, diet and exercise approaches can be developed to address the specific insulin defect involved. This would include not only whether to focus more on diet as compared to exercise, but also what type of diet and exercise program would be best. For example, a dietary approach would seem more significant as it relates to liver insulin resistance since high-fat, high-sugar diets speed the development of liver resistance.

A movement-centered approach would be more important in muscle resistance because movement alone is valuable in reducing blood sugar levels. The type of exercise has different effects on different tissues. Recent studies have shown that resistance training strongly impacts both liver resistance and peripheral resistance (i.e., muscle), while cardiovascular exercise may focus more strongly on peripheral resistance. It seems this has much to do with the type of muscle fibers engaged.

Type 1 muscle fibers are the body's endurance fibers and are involved in endurance activities like running. Since type 1 (oxidative) muscle fibers are the richest source of the glucose receptor (glut4), they are excellent at reducing resistance in the muscle tissue. Type 2 muscle fibers are involved in strength and power and are primarily activated in explosive sprinting and weight training. Type 2 (glycolytic)-dominated resistance training helps with muscle resistance as well but also has interesting effects on insulin-related genes in the liver.[21]

A February 2008 study in the journal *Cell Metabolism* showed that increasing the growth of type 2b muscle fibers has substantial and indirect effects on liver glucose metabolism.[22] This study demonstrated that changes in type 2b muscle fibers reversed insulin resistance induced on the liver by a high-fat, high-sugar diet. Of the 1,200-plus genes involved in liver insulin resistance, simply the act of stimulating type 2 muscle fibers to grow was able to impact 800 or so of these genes to revert back to normal function.

Although the mechanism is not understood, the authors specu-
lated that myokines (signaling molecules released from muscle)
might be playing a role.

Real-World Example of Managing Insulin

It is not often talked about, but there is a group of people who
have mastered the use of insulin and whose lifestyle closely
resembles the springtime construct of early man. This population
can literally burn fat at will and develop the leanest physiques in
the athletic world. This is because they use exercise and diet to
maximize insulin's muscle-building potential while minimizing
its fat-storing effects. These athletes are known as figure athletes,
and they include bodybuilders, fitness competitors, and female
figure competitors. This athletic population has been ignored
largely because of the stigma associated with their sport. The
common perception is that these athletes use performance-en-
hancing drugs. This is true of some in the professional ranks, but
there is a much larger body of figure athletes who are completely
natural. However, looking at the practices of both drug-free and
drug-using figure athletes can be instructive for understanding
the physiological action of insulin.

It is a well-established practice of drug-enhanced bodybuilders
to use exogenous insulin to promote muscle gain. Although the
goals of these individuals may be questionable, it is interesting
to note a population voluntarily increasing their insulin levels
under the influence of an environment low in fat, high in protein,
and with vigorous weight training. Contrary to what is seen with
the overweight and obese, this population is able to achieve the
leanest physique in the athletic world. Interestingly, this dual

action of insulin can be seen in type 1 diabetics who either participate in activity or do not. The latter can become obese, while the former remain lean and muscular. Both kinds of type 1 diabetics demonstrate populations whose insulin regulation is under voluntary control. It is the strong influence of each diabetic's chosen lifestyle that determines whether they will be lean or overweight. The insulin-dependent diabetic who engages in intense physical training and pays close attention to diet remains insulin sensitive, while the ones who remain sedentary and pay very little attention to food choices can and do become insulin resistant.

Insulin sensitivity is mediated by environmental influences on not just insulin but other hormones as well. It is important to remember that hormones act differently based on several factors: how much hormone is present, how sensitive the cells are to the hormone's action, and what other hormones are acting along with it. Other hormones, including glucagon, growth hormone, and sex steroids, influence insulin sensitivity as well. When insulin is in balance with other hormones, it can be influenced toward muscle building while other hormones focus on fat burning. If the lifestyle factors that induce this state could be taught to weight loss clients, the outcomes would potentially be far better than simply telling people to lower insulin levels as much as possible. As we have seen, just because insulin levels are low does not automatically mean the tissues will be insulin sensitive. It is really about regaining insulin sensitive. It's about enough, but not too much insulin.

So what does all this mean when it comes to insulin? How should we view insulin in the context of calories? A simple way to think about this is to realize that just because you are losing weight does not mean you are losing fat exclusively. Depending on the approach, you could be losing muscle as well. Clinically, I have seen traditional approaches to weight loss result in 20–40 percent loss in lean tissue as well (muscle, water, organ tissue, etc.). The reverse is also true. Just because you are gaining weight does not mean that weight is always excess fat. You could instead be gaining muscle.

Calories may be driving the weight loss or weight gain, but hormones are influencing what type of weight is lost or gained. In particular, when someone is insulin sensitive, they are more likely to lose more fat than muscle in calorie deficits and more likely to gain more muscle than normal in situations of calorie excess. This is one of the reasons sex steroids like estrogen and testosterone can aid fat loss. They influence things due to their influence on insulin sensitivity.

Insulin is a hunger hormone as well. How much of this hunger suppression is a direct effect of insulin, or simply a result of insulin's impact on leptin, is not entirely clear, but if you want to attain and maintain a calorie deficit to drive fat loss, you need to keep hunger under control. Low insulin levels or insulin resistance at the level of the brain may be the cause of increased hunger. Insulin sensitivity, having enough of a healthy insulin signal, may be a primary means to control hunger.

Insulin is not the primary driver of metabolism but rather one of a number of hormones that integrate with calorie intake to influence body composition.

The Rest of the Hormone Story

I will tackle the sex steroids (estrogen, progesterone, and testosterone) and the stress hormone cortisol in depth in coming chapters. Of course, the amount of signaling molecules in human metabolism is unfathomable. We know some, but most we don't. Rather than going on and on about all the different hormones in the body, I'll give a wide overview of the rest of the story to help you understand any hormones or other signaling molecules in context.

Remember, the metabolism is working much like a stress barometer and a thermostat. It takes the "temperature" of what is going on inside and outside of the body. It then adjusts itself up or down to account for the situation in the outside environment with the activity and needs of the cells inside of the body.

You may wonder how the body does this. Because this book is mainly about the art and science of losing fat and keeping that fat off, let's start with the fat cells. Fat cells grow under the influence of insulin and excess calories. Other hormones, like cortisol, can also get in on the action. When it comes to fat release from fat cells and fat entry into fat cells, there are two regulating enzymes. HSL (hormone-sensitive lipase) shuttles fat out of fat cells. LPL (lipoprotein lipase) shuttles fat into fat cells.

To keep this straight in your head, think of these two enzymes as bouncers at a bar: Harry (HSL) and Larry (LPL). Larry lets people in the bar and Harry kicks them out. Insulin activates Larry and deactivates Harry, meaning more people get into the bar than are leaving. Cortisol activates both Harry and Larry. So when insulin and cortisol are around together with plenty of extra calories, Larry is doubly active while Harry is more subdued. This is one of the reasons why high-calorie, sugar-rich diets combined with stress are a massive signal to store rather than release fat.

Fat Messengers

Fat cells, in addition to receiving messages from the other tissues, send a ton of different messages themselves. The hormones released from fat cells are called adipokines. These molecules leave the fat cell and tell other tissues like the brain, immune system, muscle, and liver what the body's fat stores look like. I mentioned some of these molecules above (adiponectin, resistin, TNF-alpha), but perhaps the most important fat-derived hormone is leptin.

Leptin is the body's fuel gauge hormone. As the fat cell grows under the influence of calories and insulin, leptin levels rise. Leptin leaves the fat cell and signals other parts of the metabolism how to behave. Most importantly, leptin tells the brain that the body has enough fat stored away and the brain, in response, shuts down hunger. Leptin, like insulin, provides another example of the Goldilocks rule of hormones. Shrinking fat cells and the corresponding low levels of leptin signaling the brain will increase hunger. That makes sense, right? After all, the metabolism needs a way to measure its fuel reserves to guard against starvation. The confusing thing is that the same thing happens when leptin levels are chronically high. In obesity, where leptin levels are always high, the brain becomes desensitized to leptins satiating signals. This is another case of hormone resistance, only this time with leptin. This means leptin levels that are too low or too high for too long both register as starvation to the brain. This explains why many overweight people are insatiably hungry despite having plenty of fat on their body. Leptin resistance is part of the problem.

Muscle Messengers

The fat cells are not the only cells receiving and sending signals—the muscle tissue is as well. Where fat cells release adipokines, muscle cells release myokines. Most of these "muscle molecules" are released from exercising muscle. When you move your muscle, all kinds of things begin to happen depending on the type, intensity, and duration of exercise. Like the fat cells, muscle cells need to signal to the rest of the body the demands it is under.

Let's say you are doing a mixed conditioning workout that involves weightlifting with moderately heavy weights and lots of repetitions. The rest periods between lifts are very short. This type of workout is going to cause the muscle to begin to fatigue fast. You are going to feel the weight quickly getting heavy. You'll feel mechanical strain and an increasing muscle burn, and you'll be out of breath pretty much the entire time. This all is happening because the workout is demanding a lot from your muscles.

The muscles are receiving signals from the brain primarily through nerve stimulation but also through hormonal output through the HPA axis (hypothalamus-pituitary-adrenal axis) to release adrenaline and cortisol. Those two hormones signal the liver to ramp up glycogen breakdown and also signal the fat cells to release some fat. The purpose is to give the muscles energy in the form of glucose and fats to power the movement that is required.

At the same time, as the muscles move, they are registering how much stress they are under. The mechanical strain the muscles are subjected to is one kind of stress. The metabolic demands (changes in cellular pH, free radical stress, etc.) are another kind of stress. The degree to which energy demands in the muscles are met by energy availability is another kind of stress. This stress and strain on the muscle determine how the muscle communicates to the rest of the body.

As the intensity of the exercise rises, energy production in the muscle begins to be strained. As fat and carbs are broken down for energy in the muscle (primarily carbs in the case of high-intensity exercise), they are made into a compound called acetyl-CoA. This compound enters into a biochemical "waterwheel" called the Krebs cycle. Acetyl-CoA pours into the waterwheel from above, meeting with another compound called oxaloacetate. This causes the biochemical roundabout to run through a series of reactions that strips off hydrogen ions. These hydrogen ions catch a ride on mitochondrial shuttles (NAD and FADH) and are brought into the inner mitochondria where they form a chemical/electrical gradient that kicks off the electron transport chain, a series of reactions that pass electrons like a hot potato from one protein to the next. In the final step, ATP, the energy currency of the cell, is created.

When cellular energy demands exceed the amount of oxygen and glucose that can be converted to energy fast enough (i.e., aerobic metabolism), the mitochondrial shuttles become "maxed out." This comes along with a buildup of hydrogen ions in the cell and a change in cellular pH (i.e., the cells start to become more acidic). Since all the enzymes that power cellular machinery function in a narrow pH range, this change causes fatigue, a slowdown in metabolic output, and a burning sensation in the muscle.

The metabolism buffers against this by using lactate to "grab" a proton (hydrogen ion) and become lactic acid. This buffers against the pH changes. Although many people believe lactic acid causes the burning sensation, it actually buffers against it. This shift where the mitochondrial shuttles become maxed out and lactic acid begins to form is the hallmark of anaerobic metabolism. The cell has reached its peak in aerobic capacity and adds on the anaerobic contributions to energy production.

While all of this is going on, the muscle cell begins to secrete muscle molecules (technically myokines). You can think of these molecules as "metabolic smoke." The muscle is working at a frantic capacity, and the degree of stress causes a flood of different chemicals to be generated and released.

IL-6, a signaling molecule the immune cells and fat cells also use, is increased by huge margins. This compound is normally considered an inflammatory compound because when it is released from the immune system or fat cells, it also comes along with other inflammatory compounds like IL-1 beta and TNF-alpha. However, when released from muscle, it works differently. Remember, hormones are like people and behave differently depending on whom they are socializing with. When IL-6 is released from muscle in large amounts without TNF-alpha and IL-1 beta, it instead triggers other more beneficial compounds like IL-10, which are anti-inflammatory. IL-6 also acts on the brain, liver, and fat tissue and has impacts on hunger, liver glucose release, and fat release from fat cells.

The muscle also releases compounds like IL-8 and IL-15. IL-8 signals new blood vessel growth, while IL-15 signals muscle cells to grow. Lactic acid is also a signaling molecule triggering the release of human growth hormone and ramping up mitochondrial biogenesis (i.e., the making of new mitochondria). Nitric oxide (NO) is another signaling molecule from muscle that has beneficial effects on blood vessels and acts as another mitochondrial growth primer.

The point of going through all of this is not to overwhelm you but to demonstrate that the metabolism is one big communications hub. It uses many different kinds of signaling molecules to communicate. For simplicity, I refer to all of these signaling molecules as hormones, although biochemically speaking, they are not all technically hormones. New signaling molecules and mechanisms are being discovered all the time. One study showed a previously unknown mechanism where mechanical overload on muscle from weight training caused those muscles to release vesicles containing micro-RNA.[23] These vesicles left the muscle cell, traveled to the fat cell, and resulted in the fat cell ramping up its fat-releasing activities.

FAT CELLS, THE GUT, AND ALL OTHER HORMONES

Fat cells, the immune system, and the gut are immense areas of metabolic output and signaling. Cytokines, adipokines, and myokines are signaling molecules that come from the immune system, fat tissue, and muscle cells, respectively. These molecules used to be seen as compounds that only communicated in a limited fashion—only being able to signal to other cells in close proximity. Now we know that many, if not all, of them can act on cells at distant sites in the same way traditional hormones do. This is why the bucket term "hormone" is often used to now describe all signaling molecules.

Even though each of these compartments has its own signaling molecules, they also have some overlap. For example, the interleukins (IL-1, IL-10, IL-6, IL-8, IL-15, and others) are used by the immune system, fat, and muscle. Although we often talk about the body as having different systems, we now know they are all communicating with each other all the time.

We are even beginning to see that damaged particles or extracellular DNA and RNA can act as important metabolic signals as well. DAMPs and PAMPs are another class of signaling molecule you'll want to be aware of. DAMPs is an acronym that stands for damage-associated molecular patterns. When a cell is disrupted through injury or an invading organism like a bacteria or virus, the damaged material can signal the immune system to act. These compounds are also sometimes called alarmin as they signal the alarm and usher metabolic resources to fight, rescue, respond, and recover. PAMPs are pathogen-associated molecular patterns. Basically, DAMPs and PAMPs do similar things, only one comes from damage of the body and one comes from the foreign or invading agent.

The Gut

The gut is perhaps the most important and interesting hub of signaling in the body. The gut is responsible for digesting, absorbing, and assimilating food. From the moment you look at food, smell food, or expect food, the gut goes to work. When food hits your tongue, you are not just tasting for pleasure, but rather, the metabolism is sending signals. In this case, it's known as the neurolingual response (neuro = nerve and lingual = tongue), literally the tongue's connection to the brain.

Certain flavors send certain messages. If you taste sweet, the metabolism expects sugar. Even before one drop of the sugar gets into your blood, the tongue has already communicated to the brain and the brain has already communicated to the pancreas one message: expect sugar. In response, the body begins to ramp up insulin release. This is why consuming sugar, as compared to getting the same amount through IV, elicits a greater insulin response. Other flavors have an impact as well. Umami or savory says something about amino acids. Bitter and sour may convey information about the safety of the food (i.e., Is it spoiled? Will it make us sick?).

There are seven tastes we know about in science. The traditional five tastes include sweet, salty, bitter, sour, and savory. Recently, researchers discovered that fat is another taste. In addition to sensing the texture of fat (i.e., slippery or creamy), we actually can taste fat as well (though it's not great without other flavors going along with it). The last taste is actually the absence of taste, or bland.

The neurolingual phase of digestion is an important one that is not only communicating what the metabolism might expect in terms of macronutrients (fat, carbs, and protein) but also priming the brain in other ways, some known and others not. Certain flavors and textures are extremely pleasurable for the brain and can cause us to eat more than we otherwise would by kicking off dopamine, the brain chemical of seeking reward.

Combinations of sugar, fat, salt, starch, and alcohol can cause pleasure and overeating. Bitter, sour, and bland foods can have the opposite effect. More variety of flavor or more food choices can also cause us to eat more. There is even a sensory-specific satiety. The theory here is that the brain likes to "fill up" on each flavor. This is why you could be completely full of steak and potatoes, then have a bite of dessert and feel like a whole other appetite just opened up.

As you chew the food, digestive enzymes in the mouth start to digest. Bacteria in the oral cavity also go to work on some of the food. Some of these bacteria produce signaling molecules. The bacteria in the back of the tongue, when exposed to nitrate-rich vegetables, fix the nitrate into nitrite which then becomes nitric oxide (NO). NO has many metabolic functions including signaling the smooth muscles lining blood vessels to relax and improve blood flow. Some research has shown this can aid performance. Beets and beet juices are loaded with nitrate that can easily become NO and enhance exercise performance.

As the food travels into the stomach, other enzymes are released along with hydrochloric acid. The enzymes in the stomach are primarily there for protein digestion. The hydrochloric acid helps digest protein and kill bacteria, viruses, and fungi. The stomach senses how much food is present via stretch receptors telling the brain and the rest of the digestive system what to do. Whether the stomach has food in it or not impacts the hunger hormone ghrelin. When food is in the stomach, ghrelin is turned down and hunger is reduced. The longer the stomach is empty, the more ghrelin is turned up and hunger is turned on.

When the food leaves the stomach and enters the upper small intestine, the food is mixed with bile acids from the gallbladder and pancreatic enzymes from the pancreas. The small intestine also starts to release different hormones called incretins. CCK, GLP-1, and GIP are a few of these incretins. All three signal the brain to decrease hunger. GLP-1 and GIP also communicate with the pancreas and aid insulin release.

The cells of the small intestine continue to "taste" the food you have eaten. Of course, you don't sense the flavors like you do with the tongue. These cells, known as L and K cells, instead sense the viscosity and nutrient composition of the food and then send feedback to other parts of the body about what to expect and what to do. GLP-1 and GIP both respond to carbs, fat, and protein, although GLP-1 may be more associated with protein and fat and GIP more with carbs. The ratio of activity of GLP-1 to GIP is a topic of hot debate in metabolism research. GLP-1, along with another gut hormone present further down in the digestive tract called PYY, are now suspected of playing a key role in how full we feel from a meal, how long we stay full, and how sensitive and efficient we are to digestion and insulin secretion. In fact, some of the newest drugs in obesity and diabetes use GLP-1 to their advantage. There are natural agents that do the same thing. Bitter food like black coffee and plain cocoa as well as herbal compounds like berberine may have their health benefits in part due to GLP-1 activity.

Once food hits the large intestines, it enters into one of the most fascinating areas of research in metabolism, the gut microbiome. If you are a healthcare practitioner or serious health enthusiast, you have definitely heard about the gut microbiome. Much has been said about the topic in the lay public, diet books, blogosphere, and worlds of documentaries and podcasts. The microbiome is an exciting area for sure. However, right now, science really does not have much in the way of actual interventions.

We know the microbiome is a huge hub of activity and a constant source of signaling molecules we absorb into our body. One of the most popular of these is a PAMP (pathogen-associated molecular pattern) called LPS (also known as endotoxin). LPS can trigger immune reactivity, irritate the hypothalamus, and for some individuals, cause all manner of metabolic dysfunction. The gut is also the source of other positive signaling molecules and a source of nutrition. For example, gut bacteria are a source of the short-chain fatty acid butyrate, which aids the energy needs, repair, and proper regulation of enterocytes (the cells that line the digestive tract).

Even though this is a huge topic of research, there is not much I can tell you about what this means. What we do know is that although the microbiome is very fluid, changing from day to day based on what you eat, it is also relatively stable from individual to individual over the long run. The healthiest microbiomes seem to be those with a large diversity of bacteria rather than just sheer numbers. We do know that taking probiotics does not seem to alter the microbiome in huge ways, but certain types of gut bacteria have been shown useful in certain kinds of digestive conditions.

At this point, all you really need to know is that the microbiome is a *huge* reservoir of metabolic activity and certainly impacting metabolism in powerful ways. We don't yet know how to manipulate this area beyond simply eating more fiber and consuming naturally fermented foods. All that being said, you now have the background to understand that the gut microbes are likely also contributing to metabolic signaling and impacting things like hunger, cravings, mood, and immune function.

FINAL THOUGHTS

All of this should give you some hints about where we are headed in our understanding of metabolism. These signaling molecules are the way cells and tissues in one area communicate to cells and tissues in other areas. What are they communicating? They're telling the body to be on alert. To recover or repair. To increase or decrease fat release. To switch from burning mostly sugar to mostly fat or ketones. To alert about injury or infection. To signal adaptation responses like growing muscle or repairing ligaments. To be hungry or feel full. And on and on it goes. Hormonal signaling is the music of the metabolism. The metabolism does not speak English—it speaks metabolism, and the words of that language are written by hormones.

Metabolic signaling through hormones is *everything*. And at the same time, we know only a tiny fraction of the signaling molecules at play and what they do. Many people make a lot of noise about this hormone or that hormone. There is a lot of hype and discussion every time another signaling molecule or mechanism is uncovered.

You don't need to know all these signaling molecules. Don't worry about their names, and definitely don't go chasing down complex mechanisms. As we saw with insulin, it is folly to try to make decisions off the actions of one hormone. Invariably, that hormone is going to be impacted by other hormones. For every mechanism we know, there are tens or hundreds more that modify, amplify, or negate the other.

So how do we make sense of all this, then? Biofeedback, that's how. These hormones directly or indirectly impact sensations you feel every single day. By paying attention to things like hunger, mood, energy, joint pain, digestive symptoms, cravings, headaches, libido, menses, erections, focus, motivation, skin, vision, and so forth, you have a window into your hormonal balance. In the next chapter, I am going to show you how the complicated science in this chapter can be made so simple even a child can learn to understand their metabolism.

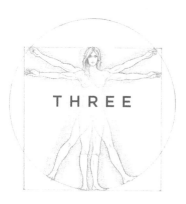

THREE

THE METABOLIC DETECTIVE

With willpower as their only tool, dieters are doomed. They might even push themselves to the brink all week, only to binge on the weekend because they desperately need a break, and in their mind, all that hard work Monday through Friday justifies a big indulgence. They don't understand that overeating on the weekend is enough to put them in a calorie excess. They don't understand how what they eat or don't eat at one meal directly impacts what they will or won't eat later. Their one tool is simply never going to be enough to get them the results they want.

Detectives, on the other hand, know they need an entire kit full of tools in order to do their job effectively. Their approach is to listen and observe and unearth the clues that will lead them to success. Detectives understand weight loss is about much more than diet and exercise. They realize movement and mindset matter just as much as meals and metabolics. They understand metabolism is speaking its own unique language to them, and they make it their mission to learn it. Detectives also understand no two cases are the same. Just as every case has a unique set of circumstances setting it apart from every other case, every person has a unique set of factors contributing to how their metabolism works. Because of this, it's critical we only look at the clues our own bodies are giving us. Becoming a detective should automatically eliminate any ideas you have about one-size-fits-all diets.

The dieter is like someone trapped in a dark room using a single flashlight to illuminate one corner and saying, "Okay, I get it. This is the whole room." A detective knows there's way more to the room that they're not aware of yet and begins to slowly explore other parts of the room. Most knowledge comes from knowing that we don't know and being willing to admit when what we think we know is wrong. Again, if you think you're doing everything right and not getting results, you are not doing everything right. Time to start exploring.

DECODING THE LANGUAGE OF METABOLISM

At its most basic, the metabolism is a sensing and responding apparatus. It accumulates information from the outside world as a way to determine what is needed to survive. It then relays this information to the cells inside the body so they can carry out the correct biochemical reactions. It is also, simultaneously, picking up signals the cells are sending and measuring and responding to their nutrient needs and energy demands as well.

Metabolism communicates using molecules that act as little messengers relaying signals back and forth. An area of the brain called the hypothalamus gathers all this information from outside and inside the body, then adjusts metabolic actions to respond and adapt. These "metabolic messengers" are called many things including incretins, prostaglandins, cytokines, myokines, adipokines, hormones, and neurotransmitters, among others. For the sake of simplicity, I refer to all signaling molecules inside and outside the body as hormones. For example, elements of food can act as signaling molecules. The bacteria living in our guts (i.e., the microbiome) send hormone-like signals into the body. And certain phytochemicals from compounds like coffee, chocolate, berries, plastics, and chemicals of industry can all impact the metabolism by sending hormone-like signals.

The metabolism picks up changes in light, temperature, and sun exposure on the skin and releases hormones to tell the cells inside the body what time of the day it is and what season of the year you are in. The mouth and tongue collect tastes and textures of food and relay that to the brain, letting it know if the food is a meaty protein source, a starch, a sugar, a creamy fat, or a combination of them all. Depending on what you are chewing, the neurolingual response (or tongue-brain connection) prepares the body to begin the early release of insulin to capture the sugar, fats, and amino acids to be burned or stored. The small intestines continue sampling food to determine how much was eaten and what kind of macronutrients are present.

Based on this information, hormones will signal you to be full faster, stay full for longer, and be prone to future cravings or not.

The metabolism turns on and off certain functions depending on the time of the day (known as circadian rhythms) and alters energy fluctuation throughout the day (or ultradian rhythm). The metabolism is constantly sensing, adjusting, sensing, responding, sensing, and changing all the time. Its major concern is keeping you in balance. It uses its hormonal software to gather the information from inside and outside the body, then integrates the information and uses hormones, once again, to instruct the cells and the body what to do next.

Anytime the body is knocked out of balance (eating too much or too little, sleeping too much or too little, exercising too much or too little, and so on), it's the metabolism's job to restore balance, and it uses a whole host of hormonal reactions to get you back to center. Stress is what knocks the metabolism out of balance; adaptive adjustments in the hormonal and cellular responses are what try to restore balance.

So how can you possibly keep track of all this information? In truth, you can't. There are thousands of hormones in the body inducing millions of biochemical reactions. You could spend your entire life trying to memorize them all and never even come close. How, then, do we make sense of metabolic function and use it to our advantage?

It's actually fairly simple. Every hormone in the body is there to help send a signal. If you pay close attention to the body, you'll start picking up on these signals. In fact, you will start seeing the sensations in your body as hormonal biofeedback. Hunger is a hormone response; energy is impacted by several different hormones; cravings are linked to brain hormones; sleep is a complex orchestration of hormonal activity; even mood is controlled by hormonal brain chemicals.

You don't need to know the names of all the hormones in the body or what they do.

All you really need to be aware of is the biofeedback sensations you are feeling. These sensations are clues to whether your hormonal system is in balance or out of balance. This is a critical point because there are two things required for sustained and lasting fat loss: calorie deficits and hormonal balance. You likely have an understanding of the calorie part of that equation, so for now, let's take a deeper look at everything that's happening with your hormones.

KEEPING IT ALL IN CHECK

Your metabolism responds to stress and sends you specific clues to show you whether it's functioning optimally or not. As a metabolic detective, you should always be looking for things that just don't seem right, and your main source of clues is your biofeedback in the form of HEC and SHMEC (pronounced "heck and shmeck"). They are easy-to-remember acronyms that help you assess hormonal balance based on several factors we've already mentioned several times in previous sections.

HEC = *hunger, energy, cravings*
SHMEC = *sleep, hunger, mood, energy, cravings*

HEC provides biofeedback you can monitor hour by hour, day by day, whereas SHMEC focuses on all the things you can track over the course of weeks and months.

Let's break down each of those elements. It's important to first understand the difference between **hunger** and **cravings**. Hunger is an emptiness or a gnawing you feel in your gut. The hunger hormone called ghrelin (which even sounds like a growl) activates your hunger when it goes up, and you feel it in your gut. However, this isn't necessarily a bad thing. It's not that you should never feel hungry; your hunger should, however, always be under control.

When hunger is out of your control, the second you sense it, you'll think, "Oh my God, I have to eat something *now*," and will most likely end up eating more than you actually need to. When it's under control, that's a great indication the metabolism is not experiencing too much stress.

Cravings, however, are felt in the head. They're the need to taste something different or do something with your mouth. They're often linked to a behavior or habit. For example, you might always need to have popcorn while you're watching a movie. Maybe you've already eaten dinner and feel completely full and satisfied, but if there's a movie on, you better believe that popcorn is in your lap. You know you are having a craving when you feel full but have a strong desire to taste something else. I often refer to this as being full from the meal but not "dessert full." Cravings can also come as a result of boredom. Or they might be directly linked to relaxation in your mind. Perhaps you believe you can't wind down after a long day without a glass of wine. These are all behaviors or habits you build that make it all the easier for cravings to creep up.

Hunger and cravings are driven by different hormones. Cravings are highly associated with cortisol, which activates the reward center in the brain and shuts down the motivation center. Estrogen and progesterone also affect cravings, as they both have receptors all over the body, including in the brain, and can manipulate things like serotonin, dopamine, and gamma-aminobutyric acid (GABA).

Energy tends to be more complex because just about everything and anything can impact it, but when it comes to food, energy mostly comes down to blood sugar. If your energy is unstable and unpredictable, it likely means you're not managing your blood sugar, which can lead to hunger and cravings as well. These three elements are inextricably linked and capable of changing quickly. For example, we know for most people, energy tends to rise in the morning, dip between 1:00 p.m. and 3:00 p.m., then rise again before falling at night.

You can look at these undulating patterns (known as the ultradian rhythm) and pay attention to how the things you eat and when you eat them impacts your energy levels throughout the day. Then you can make modifications accordingly.

You really begin to connect the dots and see the bigger picture of why your metabolism acts the way it does when you add **sleep** and **mood** to the assessment. It helps to have several days' worth of data on each. You can ask yourself, "How did I sleep during the last week?" then compare that to what you ate and when. It's also best to analyze your mood over the course of a week, as it likely doesn't change much during the course of a typical day.

When HEC and SHMEC are in check, that's a strong indication the hormones involved in fat burning and fat storage are working in your favor.

The second HEC or SHMEC is out of check, it's a strong clue your hormones are out of balance and your metabolism is under stress. Although HEC and SHMEC can offer you valuable qualified insight into your own metabolism, their power doesn't end there. When I use the term "SHMEC," I am referring to sleep, hunger, mood, energy, and cravings, but I also use this term as a catchall phrase for all hormonal biofeedback. SHMEC also includes exercise performance and exercise recovery.

It also is an indication of hormone function that impacts reproductive capacity. If SHMEC is a barometer of stress load on the body, then reproductive function is a key aspect of SHMEC as well. After all, the prime directive of metabolism is to keep you alive long enough to reproduce and spread your genes. If there is too much stress, the metabolism will protect its reproductive resources and you will see negative changes in libido, menses, and erections.

Digestion is another major hub of metabolic activity. The brain is the command-and-control center of metabolism, and the gut is the major site of integration between the nervous system, immune system, and hormone system (the neuro-endocrine-immune system).

Finally, signs and symptoms of disease are also part of SHMEC. This can include anything from skin breakouts to joint pain, headaches to metabolic dysfunction. All biofeedback falls under SHMEC, which ultimately is a tangible way to easily assess the body's stress load, hormonal function, and metabolic balance.

HEC and SHMEC are how you read your body's stress barometer. When HEC and SHMEC are in check, you can be relatively confident that your metabolism is stable, balanced, and happy.

SHMEC IS ALL BIOFEEDBACK

While SHMEC is an acronym for some of the more important hormonal biofeedback sensations, it is also used as a catchall phrase for all hormonal feedback sensations in the body, including:

 Sleep
Tells about stress hormone and growth hormone balance. Melatonin should rise at night. Poor sleep quality or quantity creates excess cortisol and insulin.

 Hunger
Tells about hormones like CCK, PYY, GIP, and GLP-1 as well as brain insulin sensitivity.

 Mood
Balance of brain chemicals. Serotonin for relaxed self-assurance. Dopamine for drive and focus. GABA for calm steadiness. The gut plays a big role. Sex hormones matter here too.

 Energy
Stress hormone and insulin balance. Integration with neurotransmitters. Impacted by thyroid function.

 Cravings
Cortisol lowers motivation and raises reward centers in the brain. Fluctuating sex hormones indirectly impact brain.

 Exercise Performance
The ability to perform at a high level from workout to workout day after day as well as be motivated to exercise is tied closely to hormonal balance, fuel reserves, and nutrient status.

 Exercise Recovery
The ability to recover from exercise tells about fuel reserves, nutrient status, and how well the body can go from stress to recovery, relaxation, and regeneration. It also includes the balance between anabolic hormones (testosterone, estrogen, HGH) and catabolic hormones (cortisol, adrenaline, etc.).

 Digestion
The digestive system tells us how well the sympathetic and parasympathetic systems are working.

 Libido/Erection
Sexual desire and performance tell how well the body is responding to long-term stress. A chronically stressed physiology does not prioritize reproduction.

 Menses
Changes in menstrual timing, flow, and symptoms tell about balance of sex hormones.

When they are not in check, it is an indication the metabolism is compensating, becoming more rigid, and putting the brakes on fat loss. When HEC or SHMEC goes out of check, ask yourself, "What am I eating (or not eating) that's causing this? How am I sleeping? Am I actively taking steps to reduce metabolic stress? Why is this happening?" When you take the time to really pay attention, you can easily draw conclusions and make smart choices.

DIGGING EVEN DEEPER

Although HEC and SHMEC are inherently subjective, there also are newer, more advanced and objective ways you can measure stress on your metabolism and its ability to adapt, including heart rate variability and continuous glucose monitoring, among others (more on those two later). In addition, your own body measurements and weight provide clues to whether your metabolism is functioning properly. Optimal body composition and easy fat loss are consequences of hormonal balance. More importantly, they are indications that you are achieving the other half of the fat loss equation—calorie deficits. Many people argue about the number of calories needed to lose fat. The truth is, there is only one way to know for sure you have achieved a calorie deficit, and that's weight loss.

By now, you understand that either too few or too many calories can cause stress on the system. If you consume too few calories, your body thinks it's starving and holds on to fat stores. If you consume too many calories, your body thinks winter must be coming and it stores more fat. To get the body to release its fat stores requires convincing it that it has enough food not to starve and not so much food that it needs to store.

It's about achieving the Goldilocks zone—not too much, not too little, but just right—and using some of the following more advanced technology can help you get there.

HEART RATE VARIABILITY

Heart rate variability (HRV) measures the flexibility of the heart. More specifically, it measures the balance between the two sides of the nervous system: the stress reactive side (sympathetic nervous system) and the stress adaptive side (parasympathetic nervous system). Most people think the heart beats like a rigid metronome, making a rhythmic "lub-dub" sound at the same pace with the same frequency. In reality, a healthy heart is more like a symphony than a static drum, and the more it changes frequency, the healthier the metabolism. If you have too much sympathetic reactivity, it's like having an erratic conductor who loses the rhythm and causes the symphony to sound dull and repetitive. A great conductor is calm, relaxed, and Zen-like, producing music that is sophisticated, improvisational, and harmonious. HRV devices measure the music of the heart and tell you if you're under too much stress. We've all had days when we feel like working out is about the last thing we want to do. Then we go to the gym and have the best workout of our lives. We've also had days when we feel great but have the worst workout. HRV helps us understand these paradoxical times by picking up the imbalances created by stress long before we can sense the biofeedback. You might be feeling great, but if your HRV is trending down, it's an indication you are not recovering from stress well. If you don't heed this warning, you may find that SHMEC goes out of check and fat loss stalls or weight gain ensues. It is a powerful objective tool to have in your arsenal.

HRV has some weaknesses and it is not a tool you want to use in isolation. In time, though, you will begin to see how HRV relates to SHMEC and hormonal metabolic balance. You can think of it as an early warning signal like the tire pressure sensor in your car.

You can still drive your car with low tire pressure, but if you ignore it completely, you are going to have a blowout and be sidelined.

Thanks to technology, measuring HRV is as easy as downloading an app that can sense it from the touch of your finger. Or you can go with some of the fancier devices available for a range of prices at various sites online. There are now rings, wrist straps, even beds that will measure and monitor HRV. I check my HRV every day to help me determine how hard I should go with my own workouts. Exercise is a great tool to help metabolism gain and maintain flexibility. At the same time, exercise can easily be overdone and become a stress to the system. HRV can help us understand how to better balance training and recovery. For most people, an exercise program is seen as something that is the same for everyone. It is treated like a recipe. If your program calls for five days a week, that's what you do. If the protocol dictates a certain intensity to follow, that's what you adhere to. This is problematic as we are all unique with different tendencies toward overtraining and variations in time needed to recover.

A simple way to think about using HRV to easily balance training output with training recovery is to divide your workouts into red, yellow, and green days. It's like a traffic light: red is stop, yellow is take it easy, and green is go. Red is a scheduled off day, but it can also be a day you decide to take off because your SHMEC and

HRV are not trending in the right direction. On red days, you are doing very little or perhaps nothing at all. I like to use these days for light mobility work, stretching, and active recovery like yoga (only the very relaxing kind), tai chi, hiking, or walking. Sauna, contrast hydrotherapy, sleeping in, naps, meditation, sex and cuddling, and other rest and recovery activities are great on red days.

Yellow days will be the most valuable and most frequent. Yellow is a scheduled training day. You know you have a workout, and it looks exactly like what you have planned on paper.

In this case, SHMEC and HRV may be showing signs of issues and you just want to make sure you are not going to throw yourself into a metabolic tailspin by overdoing it. Remember, both too little and too much training can cause problems for metabolic health and flexibility. On a yellow day, you will do the prescribed workout but adjust the intensity to a lower level than the workout instructs. You can accomplish this with lower weights, decreased volume (i.e., lower sets and/or reps), and/or longer rest periods between sets. One of my favorite and most recommended strategies for a yellow day involves only closed-mouth breathing. By allowing yourself to breathe only through the nose, intensity and nervous system stimulation are naturally regulated. This is also a great tool for training adaptations. Nasal breathing produces more nitric oxide (NO) compared to mouth breathing and teaches the body to become more efficient at oxygen and carbon dioxide exchange in the tissues. Translation? Yellow days using nasal breathing will bolster performance on green days and competitions. All these adjustments decrease the stress on the nervous system and reduce pressure on the metabolic stress barometer. Yellow workouts are scaled back to manage metabolic balance.

Green days mean the workout is done as prescribed and perhaps with even more intensity, higher volume, shorter rest, and greater loads. Green days may even turn into all-out efforts where you are attempting personal records. These workouts are where you really challenge the metabolism to perform at its top function and are exceptionally healthy for metabolic function, provided they are not overdone.

Although biofeedback is always important to tap into, HRV gives a more objective guide to your capacity to recover. It allows you to more accurately judge the appropriateness of a green versus yellow day. If my HRV is great and I'm also feeling good (i.e., HEC and SHMEC are in check), I am likely going green that day. If my HRV is trending downward but I'm still feeling good, it's likely a yellow day.

If HRV is low and I'm not feeling good, I'm definitely opting for yellow or probably going red and taking the day off for active recovery. Often, red days are scheduled and should be taken whenever they appear on the training schedule, but HRV tells you whether you are having too many greens and not enough reds. Once you master this, you start to see increased performance in the gym, more stable SHMEC, and less fatigue, hunger, and cravings.

CONTINUOUS GLUCOSE MONITORING

Continuous glucose monitoring is another real-time tool we can use to assess stress on metabolism; it involves a small electrode placed under the skin taking regular samples of blood sugar. These devices are not technically measuring the blood but

MANAGING WORKOUT INTENSITY AND RECOVERY

Intensity of workouts:

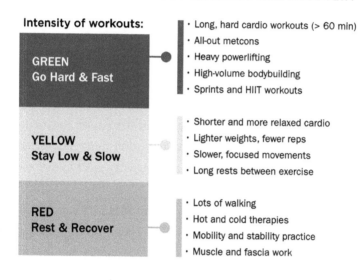

GREEN
Go Hard & Fast

- Long, hard cardio workouts (> 60 min)
- All-out metcons
- Heavy powerlifting
- High-volume bodybuilding
- Sprints and HIIT workouts

YELLOW
Stay Low & Slow

- Shorter and more relaxed cardio
- Lighter weights, fewer reps
- Slower, focused movements
- Long rests between exercise

RED
Rest & Recover

- Lots of walking
- Hot and cold therapies
- Mobility and stability practice
- Muscle and fascia work

Suggested distribution:

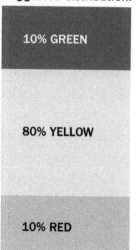

10% GREEN

80% YELLOW

10% RED

Hints:

- Red days and green days should be roughly equal.
- Green days are great days for timed workouts.
- Yellow days are great days for light volume-based workouts.
- Breathing only through the nose assures you stay yellow.
- Nasal breathing is impossible on green days.
- Go for personal records on green days.
- Perfect the moves on yellow days.
- Correlate with heart rate variability (HRV) if desired.
- Stick to your training schedule. Adjust intensity, volume, and load to turn green days yellow and yellow days green as required.

rather glucose concentrations in the interstitial space around cells, but this is highly correlated with blood levels. This helps you make the connection between low energy or intense cravings and blood sugar peaks and dips. In coming years, lasers may be able to read blood glucose levels from a simple wrist strap or ring. In fact, technology is exploding so much in the areas of both HRV and continuous glucose monitoring with wearable devices, apps, and other advances that a good metabolic detective needs to be on the lookout for anything they can add to their tool kit.

It takes a few days to see averages and trends in HRV and from continuous glucose monitoring. From that point on, any fluctuation outside of your average gives you a deeper understanding of how your metabolism is managing stress. As you become healthier and your metabolism becomes more flexible, those averages will begin to change, balance will be achieved, and HEC and SHMEC will become more stable.

If this all seems like too much work, it's okay to just stick to what works for you (that's the only rule of mastering metabolism, remember?). HEC and SHMEC are the ultimate tools to measure metabolic response.

But also paying attention to how your clothes fit may be enough for you—that's still a deeper assessment than just stepping on the scale. Maybe you like to take selfies. Use them to analyze the changes you're seeing in your body. One quick waist measurement can tell you more than ten trips to the scale. Find the tool you think works best, and use it.

MEASURING UP

Assessing weight loss only by the scale is the one-size-fits-all tool dieters just love. Metabolic detectives, on the other hand, know weight loss is about much more than a number on a scale. They know they can lose water weight and muscle as well as fat, and they use their skills to determine which one they're losing. They measure their body and track how it's changing. They measure the circumference of their waist, which is important in both men and women as it's not a very heavily muscled area and mostly filled with fat. They pay attention to how their clothes fit and how their shape has changed.

The shape of male and female physiques is one of the more valuable tools to assess to determine fat loss versus weight loss. Research has determined the healthiest body shapes for both men and women. These shapes are not just indicative of a flexible vital metabolism but also tend to be the most attractive physiques. The waist-to-chest ratio of a male is a key indicator of health and reproductive vigor, and those romantically drawn to men subconsciously assess this shape on men. Men tend to want the V-shape, with broad shoulders and a slimmer waist, that women equate with virility. Men also rate other men with this shape as more powerful and tend to prefer the same look on their own physique. The female shape is even more nuanced. For women, the shape that is healthiest and found to be most desirable by others (and the woman herself) is the hourglass shape. This is a physique where the waist-to-chest and waist-to-hip ratios approximate each other. Female models, whether plus-size, petite, or tall and thin, all tend to have this hourglass shape in common.

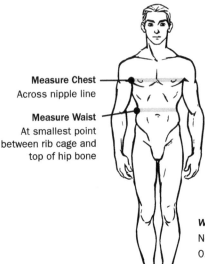

Measure Chest
Across nipple line

Measure Waist
At smallest point
between rib cage and
top of hip bone

Waist to Chest Ratio (WCR)
Normal is between 0.7–0.8,
0.77 is optimal

V-Shape
WCR is below 0.8

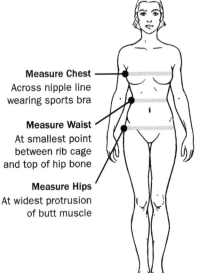

Measure Chest
Across nipple line
wearing sports bra

Measure Waist
At smallest point
between rib cage
and top of hip bone

Measure Hips
At widest protrusion
of butt muscle

Waist to Chest Ratio (WCR)
Normal is between 0.6–0.9,
0.7 is optimal

Waist to Hip Ratio (WHR)
Normal is between 0.6–0.9,
0.7 is optimal

Hourglass Shape
WCR and WHR both are
approximately equal,
optimal is 0.7 for each

From a strictly biological standpoint, the hourglass shape denotes female reproductive ability (again, this does not mean a woman has to be extremely thin to be attractive—the hourglass shape is appealing on every body frame regardless of size).

THE WEIGHT OF THE SCALE

Using the scale in addition to all of your other tools is okay. However, I know some people would rather step on broken glass than the scale. The scale can be a slippery slope, but when it's just one of the many tools in your kit, it becomes much easier to navigate.

If the scale doesn't bother you, I encourage you to weigh yourself first thing in the morning and again right before bed. That will allow you to see how your weight fluctuates during the day. For example, it is impossible to gain five pounds of fat over the weekend. It's very possible, however, to gain five pounds of water. So when you see that number eventually drop back down, you know that's not fat you're losing. It's just one more way your metabolism is speaking to you.

If, however, you find that the scale only stresses you out, skip it. Remember the law of individuality, and use another tool that is better suited for you. To be a metabolic detective, you will inevitably have to assess body composition and hormones, but the scale doesn't have to be part of that.

AIM FOR METABOLIC UNDERSTANDING

The most common tool people associate with detectives is the magnifying glass. It helps them see what the naked eye misses. It reveals things most observers would easily overlook. As a metabolic detective, you also have a tool that can help you dig deeper into what the clues are telling you—a process I call AIM.

AIM stands for **assess, investigate**, and **modify**. Your ability to do all three will allow you to better decode the language of metabolism and decipher every clue it sends your way.

Assess

When it comes to assessing, you want as much data as you can get—more data allows you to understand more of the story. A detective who walks into a murder scene is aware of every single detail. They pay attention to the position of the body, the presence of any blood, whether there are any bullet casings, and so forth. They pay attention and pinpoint certain details that simply seem off.

For the metabolic detective, this means paying particular attention to the things I've already encouraged you to look for: the 4Ps of metabolic individuality and 4Ms of metabolism. You will want to always keep these frameworks in mind as you begin the work of constructing a lifestyle that works for you. Let's cover these briefly one more time so you can see how to use them effectively when conducting your assessment.

The **4Ms of metabolism** consist of the different areas you will want to focus on. Mindfulness/mindset is about stress management. Because your metabolism acts as one big stress barometer, you need something acting as a release valve for the pressure that builds up. Mindfulness is about all the things that remove us from the daily grind and instead connect us to our center. This can include:

- Slow rhythmic movements such as walking and tai chi, yin yoga (not intense yoga), and mobility stretching
- Self-myofascial release
- Massage
- Sleep
- Meditation
- Relaxing music
- Creative pursuits
- Time spent in nature
- Water and sweat therapies
- Cuddling with pets
- Social connection
- Sex, masturbation, and orgasm
- Reading
- And others

Movement is about your pattern of daily activities. Remember, this is not exercise but rather everything you do to get things done in your day. Getting from point A to point B for ancestral humans took a lot of walking. Your metabolic software is tuned to that reality. If you are sitting and not moving during your day, your metabolism is going to remain rigid. Think of a pool of water versus a flowing stream. Water that sits will collect a layer of film and sludge. Water that flows remains clean and pure. Your body is mostly water. Sitting is the equivalent of stagnant, dirty water. Would you rather be the rusty Tin Man or have hydrated, flexible tissues?

Meals and metabolics (exercise) are the rest of the equation, but if you are the typical human, you have already overestimated these two elements. Many people think these are the most important, whereas for most, they are actually far less important than mindfulness and movement. When it comes to meals and metabolics, too much or too little is not a good thing. You need enough but not too much.

As part of your personal metabolism assessment, you should be regularly ranking each of these four elements on a scale from one to ten with the goal of achieving a six or better for each. Give yourself a ten if you are doing recovery mindfulness practices multiple times daily. Give yourself a ten on movement if you are getting between 10,000 and 20,000 steps daily. If you are getting less than 5,000 steps, score yourself with a one or two. If, on the other hand, you are getting excessive movement—above 20,000 steps daily—and not getting results, you may want to consider reducing your movement. The sweet spot seems to be between 10,000 and 20,000 steps daily.

When it comes to meals, the scoring is not as easy, but doing so can help create the personal dietary plan that works for you. I suggest you rank your adherence to your chosen meal plan. One means you are not adherent or consistent at all; ten means you are completely adherent and consistent. Once you are at an eight or better and still not getting results, that tells you either you are following a plan not beneficial for your metabolism or one of the other Ms is more important for you.

Metabolics is about exercise (it also includes things that move the metabolism like drugs and supplements). Exercise is incredibly tricky as there is a fine line between enough and too much. If you are doing everything right with the other Ms, then three times per week of intense exercise should be all most people need.

The **4Ps of metabolic individuality** include your physiology, psychology, personal preferences, and practical circumstances. You need to understand how your body responds to certain things compared to others. Perhaps running makes you hungrier and works against you rather than for you. Or maybe you have an exaggerated insulin response when you eat carbohydrates or suffer from a hidden intolerance to certain foods like dairy or wheat. These are important things to know about your physiology. Your assessment of your unique physiology will be an ongoing lifelong process. You want to begin accumulating as much information about your unique biochemistry as you can starting now.

Psychology is really about your unique way of dealing with the stresses of life. How do you respond when you are under a deadline at work? What happens when you are in an argument with your significant other? How do social interactions impact your ability to live a healthy lifestyle? These personality elements are important. For example, I grew up in a big Italian family. This means I view social situations as a time to eat and also see food as a form of love.

I have a tendency to want to finish everything on my plate and experience relaxation when I eat my favorite comfort food, pasta. These are important psychological tendencies I understand about myself. Not paying attention to how I manage food around stress and people would be a huge mistake.

Personal preferences and practical circumstances are also critical. Preferences are simply the things you love versus the things you hate. Imagine trying to live a lifestyle where you had to eat and exercise in a way that you found to be agonizing and difficult. It would not be realistic, would it? Likewise, your practical circumstances matter, even beyond your access to fresh, healthy food. It's about whether there are walking trails near you, whether you have help keeping a neat and orderly home, if you travel frequently, if you're on your feet all day, if you work sporadic shifts. All of this matters and may necessitate having a plan A, B, and C rather than just a plan A for different realities or times of the week or year.

Structured Flexibility

Admittedly, all this recording will be a pain for a lot of people in the beginning, but it will get easier over time, and after just a few days, it will help you start to make connections you likely never noticed before.

To make tracking easier, simply look for opportunities to pay closer attention as you go about your average day. We all know what it's like to overeat at a particular meal and feel terrible afterward. As a metabolic detective, if you overindulge, that's a chance for you to get to the bottom of why you did that. You can look back at the whole day (or last night and the previous day) and see what might have impacted your choice. Was it the four hours of sleep you got the night before? Was it because you didn't get enough protein at breakfast?

Was it the high stress or excessive workout you had yesterday? Clues will begin to emerge, and soon the mystery of your metabolism will be solved.

THE METABOLIC JOURNEY

HEALTH & FITNESS STRUGGLE

- DESIRE TO LOOK GOOD, FEEL GOOD, FUNCTION BETTER, LIVE LONGER

4 Ms OF METABOLISM

- MINDFULNESS
- MOVEMENT
- MEALS
- METABOLICS
- DIAGNOSIS OF WHAT THE BLOCKS TO SUCCESS ARE

AWARENESS

4 Ps OF METABOLIC INDIVIDUALITY

- PHYSIOLOGY
- PSYCHOLOGY
- PERSONAL PREFERENCE
- PRACTICAL CIRCUMSTANCES
- AN INDIVIDUAL PRESCRIPTION BASED OFF OF THE 4MS

ACTIONS AND CHOICES

THE AIM PROCESS

- ASSESS
- INVESTIGATE
- MODIFY
- THE METABOLIC DETECTIVE PROCESS
- IS SHMEC IN CHECK?
- FAT LOSS?
- VITALS?

ADJUST ACTIONS AND CHOICES

METABOLIC MODIFICATIONS

- ABSORB WHAT IS USEFUL
- DISCARD WHAT IS NOT
- ADD WHAT IS UNIQUE TO YOU
- INCORPORATE PURPOSE

REPEAT

START

There is no question the assess step of the AIM process is the most complicated. There's a lot of data to take in, and at first, you might feel a little overwhelmed. Thankfully, there's a concept called structured flexibility that will make getting started much easier than you might think it will be.

The idea behind structured flexibility is that you can start *anywhere you want*. Maybe you recently watched a documentary on veganism and you just feel compelled to give it a try. Go for it. Maybe you've always suspected that knowing more about your blood sugar could help you get a better handle on your health. Head to the pharmacy and get a monitor. Maybe something as simple as a FitBit will get you up and moving on a regular basis. Maybe you've always wanted to try keto or intermittent fasting (more on these in Chapter Ten). Whatever you choose to do becomes your structure, and once you commit to it, you become a living, breathing evidence-based science experiment. Then all you have to do is determine if the choice you made is working for you. As a metabolic detective, all the data you gain from each choice you make will be added to your tool kit until you find the lifestyle that's best for you.

Dieters mistakenly think the process stops with structure. They become so obsessed with meal plans, recipes, and someone else telling them what to do that they never bother to do the work to find out what really works for *them*. Metabolic detectives know structure is only a blueprint—something to work with in the beginning. Your personal experience will determine what you end up building as much as that blueprint. This is where the flexibility comes in. You will continue to monitor your HEC and SHMEC, measure your body composition, inspect your vitals/

blood labs, and do all the things we've covered in this chapter, and if everything is in check, the choices you have made are the right ones for you.

Investigate

With the data from the assess part in hand, take a step back and ask, "What's working and what isn't?" If HEC and SHMEC are in check and you're losing fat, you know your metabolism is responding. That's the holy grail. All you have to do is avoid the temptation to try to do more. That's what a dieter would do, but metabolic detectives know better than to try and speed up the process. Don't try to cut out more calories. Don't start going crazy with exercise. Remember, you don't want a fast metabolism; you want a flexible metabolism. The metabolism works best in the Goldilocks zone, and if you have just found it, hold that position and ride that wave until it stops working, then readjust when necessary.

If, however, HEC and SHMEC are in check but you're not losing fat, don't despair. You're already winning the hardest part of the battle. Now is when you can begin to decrease calories. It's best to push your energy intake down with diet rather than exercise, as most people don't respond to exercise the way they want and you could easily throw off your metabolism. Again, how you cut out calories is up to you. You could cut your carbohydrate intake, cut your fat amounts, or focus on calories from both. Maybe you want to start tracking your intake, or perhaps you wish to take a more intuitive approach. Whatever you choose to do is fine in this scenario because the metabolism is in a position of strength. As long as the hormones are balanced, indicated by a strong and stable HEC and SHMEC, you are safe to push on the metabolism with lower energy intake to entice it to use its own fat stores for energy.

On the other hand, you could find you are losing fat, but HEC and SHMEC are out of whack. Now you're on a slippery slope. You have officially entered the dieter's trap, where it *seems* like everything you want to happen is happening, but it's an illusion. Your metabolism is going to compensate.

It's like a boomerang—the harder you throw it, the faster it's going to whip right back at your head. You have to get HEC and SHMEC in check or else you will suffer what I call the metabolic credit card effect, short-term gain with long-term penalties.

The most important part of the investigation part of this process is to develop a keen sense of observation. Really try to understand how your choices and decisions around diet, exercise, and lifestyle are leading to changes that may or may not serve you. All you really need to do is categorize your results into the four different outcomes we just discussed:

- SHMEC in check and losing fat
- SHMEC in check and not losing fat or gaining fat
- SHMEC not in check and losing fat
- SHMEC not in check and not losing fat or gaining fat

Once you are clear on which of these outcomes you find yourself in, you are ready to modify your approach to get you to a place where SHMEC is in check and you are attaining or maintaining optimal body composition.

Modify

By now, the first two steps of the AIM process have revealed to you how your approach to food impacts your hormones and, in turn, your HEC and SHMEC. This might mean you're now realizing the way you've been doing things up to this point isn't really doing you any favors. The last step of the process—modify—is a way of making sure your new approach is as balanced as possible.

Let's address this by seeing how you may want to modify your approach based on two of the possible outcomes of the investigation phase.

SHMEC in Check and Fat Loss

As we discussed previously, this is exactly where you need to be. It is the only sustainable outcome in the process of fat loss and body change. This outcome indicates you have achieved the two things required for fat loss: hormonal metabolic balance (i.e., SHMEC in check) and calorie deficits. The calorie deficit leads to weight loss; the hormonal balance controls hunger and cravings while ensuring the weight you do lose is coming mostly from fat. In this scenario, there is absolutely nothing at all to modify. You simply keep doing exactly what you are doing. Also, keep in mind that the nature of metabolism is to change, so eventually, you will slip out of this state and need to rework the process to find it once more.

SHMEC Not in Check with Fat Loss

As discussed, this is a tricky place to be. It may feel like this is a great place to be, but it is actually a warning sign. The fact that SHMEC is out of check means your hormonal system is priming you to regain all the weight you may have lost and then some.

Remember, 95 percent of dieters regain the weight, while 66 percent end up fatter as a result of going on a diet. This is the scenario that causes it, and you must work hard to quickly modify your dietary approach to avoid this negative outcome.

At this point, I recommend a five-step process to get HEC back in check. You should work through these five stages one meal or one day at a time.

Step 1: Increase lean protein, fiber, and water to curb hunger and suppress cravings. The amino acids in protein, as well as the meaty texture of some protein sources, slow down digestion and signal to the brain that it has enough nutrients and can stop being so hungry. The goal is to provide maximum hunger suppression with minimal calories. Foods rich in protein, fiber, and water but scarce in fat and starch easily accomplish this.

Think of foods like boneless skinless chicken breasts, egg whites, leafy greens, low-starch vegetables, and low-sugar fruits like berries, apples, and pears, as well as plenty of water as a beverage or included in foods (many vegetables and fruits make up the most water-rich food items). There is certainly nothing wrong at all with starch and fat, but as a detective, you want to know how different food elements impact your individual biochemistry. Separating out food items can help you accomplish that. A great way to think of this step is to simply turn to low-starch and low-fat soups, salads, scrambles, shakes, and stir-fries. These meals are rich in protein, fiber, and water and can be used at the next meal to get HEC back in check or substituted in at the appropriate meal the next day. Also, drinking more plain water in between meals, during meals, and right before meals is a great way to suppress hunger.

Step 2: Add some fat—any kind of fat. If protein, fiber, and water additions don't work, the next step is to add fat on top of those additions. At this step, you are still keeping the additional protein, fiber, and water but also adding a bit of fat to a meal or meals. How much fat? One tablespoon of oil, butter, or any other type of fat will do. One tablespoon is around nine grams and around 100 calories. Fat, like protein and fiber, can help some people control hunger by decreasing the speed of digestion and releasing certain hunger hormones like CCK.

Step 3: Take out the fat and add in starch. Here, you leave in the added protein, fiber, and water but sub in carbohydrates instead of fat. Again, there is nothing wrong with starch or fat. The point of this exercise is to determine if carbohydrates are more satiating and satisfying for you than fat. This is an extremely valuable thing for you to discover about your unique physiology. You always want to gather as much information about your reactions to macronutrients as possible. How much do you add? Think in terms of bites. A tablespoon of rice, oats, or potato is about ten grams by weight and contains about eight grams of carbohydrate and thirty calories.

This is not exact, but it is a good rule of thumb. Three to four bites of starch are about 100 calories and twenty-five grams of carbs.

Step 4: Add both starch and fat. If the process of separating out starch and fat is not working, then adding both together is the next thing to try. Here, you are adding a serving of fat as well as a serving of starch. This combination can be a potent hunger-suppressing aid and crave-reducing agent. It also will quickly amplify the calories in a meal.

Step 5: Add a meal or a snack. If none of the above works to control hunger, energy, and cravings, then adding a strategically placed meal is the next thing to do. If you tend to be excessively hungry or craving at lunch, this meal would be best placed mid-morning between breakfast and lunch. Most individuals in the Western world tend to eat their largest number of calories at night. They also tend to be prone to excessive hunger in the hours between lunch and dinner. A small snack around 3:00 p.m. or 4:00 p.m. could be the trick to reduce excessive dinner and nighttime hunger.

My clinical experience suggests this approach is ideal for figuring out what's throwing your hormones off track. Research also suggests that individualizing dietary approaches is more successful than one-size-fits-all strategies. A good metabolic detective will use both personal experience and research in their process of discovery. It is important to remember that research is a tool for averages, not individuals. You can certainly use research as a means to get you in the ballpark, but there is no escaping this process if you really want to master your individual metabolic understanding.

You might already know fat is important for you to control your hunger. After all, there's nothing wrong with fat if it offers you a benefit (there's actually no such thing as "wrong" when you're trying to determine how different things affect your individual metabolism). So skip that step.

There's also no specific time element dictating when you should do each step. You can do them meal by meal, day by day, or a combo of both. In the meal-by-meal scenario, you adjust your next meal based on the response from your previous meal. If breakfast left you with HEC out of check, you would make corrections at the very next meal. In the day-by-day situation, you would alter the same meal the next day. For example, I might wake up and eat my normal breakfast of two eggs over-medium, oatmeal, and some berries. If I'm ravenous by lunch and wolf down a burger and fries, I clearly need to adjust my breakfast the next day. This is a great time to introduce some protein, fiber, and water, so I might add another egg the following morning. It's best to eat your protein, fiber, and water first in the meal for two reasons: (1) doing so leads to better blood sugar regulation, and (2) you don't need to always eat everything on your plate. Protein, fiber, and water are most likely to get HEC in check, so they get top priority, and you may find yourself full and satisfied, leaving some calories behind.

Now you can move to the next step. Maybe adding that extra egg did not completely correct HEC. You can add some butter to introduce some fat and see what effect that has on your hunger and cravings. Then you can take away the butter and add more oats. Next, try a small amount of both. Finally, if none of that works, try a handful of almonds halfway between breakfast and lunch as a small snack. Each step should reveal something new to you and give you more insight into how your metabolism is working throughout the day. It might take a week to work through the entire process, but by the end of it, you'll know exactly what meals are most capable of keeping your HEC and SHMEC happy.

Although this might seem like a pain in the beginning, after a few weeks, your intuition will be trained to automatically know what works and what doesn't. Intuition is a skill that requires practice, and there's no such thing as intuition without experience. Think about Captain Sully, the pilot who successfully landed a plane on the Hudson River in 2009 after both engines went down, saving 155 people. Sully's intuition told him he couldn't get back to the airport despite everyone telling him he could. The thousands and thousands of hours he spent in the air up to that moment let him know the river was the safer landing spot. His experience informed his intuition, and he listened.

You can't have intuition around food if you've never practiced paying attention to what you're eating, how much you're eating, and the effect it has on you. Digging deep into HEC and SHMEC will give you the experience you need to fine-tune your intuition.

If you need more convincing, consider the following examples and how they used all of the data to get real results.

THE AIM PROCESS

 1 ASSESS
IS SHMEC IN CHECK?
Sleep/Hunger/Mood/Energy/Cravings

DID YOU LOSE FAT?
Weight/Circumference/Fat

 2 INVESTIGATE
POSSIBLE SCENARIOS

1. SHMEC in check, fat lost.
2. SHMEC in check, fat NOT lost.
3. SHMEC NOT in check, fat lost.
4. SHMEC NOT in check, fat NOT lost.

 3 MODIFY
ADJUST BASED ON SCENARIOS ABOVE

1. DO NOTHING.
2. Reduce cals and/or adjust macros.
3. Get SHMEC in check. Raise protein, fiber, and water.
4. Get SHMEC in check. Raise protein, fiber, and water. Lower fat/starch. Track cals.

Example 1: Jane

Jane, age thirty-three, just watched a documentary on a plant-based, vegetarian diet. She is excited and motivated by what she saw and is now seeking my advice for help with weight loss. I explain to her that a plant-based vegetarian diet is an amazing place to start and that her metabolism will tell us if this is the correct approach for her or not. In this case, Jane has already chosen her structure. She is going to follow a quality over quantity approach by eating a vegan diet and forgoing any animal products. We talk about how many times a day she eats. She is used to eating meals plus snacks and eats four to six times daily. Again, I tell her this structure is fine and we will soon see if it is indeed working.

Jane starts out at 5' 4" and about 170 pounds. She is muscular and tends to store most of her fat around her midsection. We use her waist circumference and body weight as our measures of progress. Her waist starts at thirty-four inches.

After the first week, she returns. Remember, we are looking for two things. First, we want her hormonal balance to remain balanced and stable. This means we want her HEC and SHMEC in check. After inquiring, we find that she is having significant hunger and cravings. We also find that her weight has gone up just slightly and her waist measurement is the same.

My first recommendation is always to get HEC and SHMEC in check first.

So we need to go back to our five-step process. Given Jane is a vegan, the first recommendation of adding more protein, fiber, and water turns into mostly a fiber and water recommendation. We add two cups of berries to her morning routine of cream of rice and banana. We also suggest oat bran instead of the cream of rice. We add a large salad at lunch and dinner and switch her bread to high-fiber bread.

When she returns the following week, she is dealing with the same issues. Hunger and cravings are problematic, and she still has not lost any weight, although she is no longer gaining. After a long chat about the need for adequate protein, Jane agrees to add eggs and dairy to her vegan diet. We now add in a vegetable scramble and whey protein smoothies at breakfast. We also add a protein smoothie when she returns home from work to help with her hunger, which is worse at night.

On follow-up, her HEC and SHMEC are largely in check, but we still have no fat loss. Because we've been using the intuitive approach, it's now time to start tracking food. She finds this stressful and daunting, so we hold off and instead focus on ways we can decrease her calories intuitively. We find she is frequently snacking on nuts at night, so we make the switch to something lower calorie like popcorn. This seems to do the trick. Her HEC and SHMEC stay in check, and at the next visit, we see fat loss. This lasts another three weeks, and she ends up losing about three pounds and an inch off her waist before things stall. Once again, we work the process. In the end, we find Jane does best on a pescatarian diet lower in fat and higher in carbohydrates. She ends up losing twenty-five pounds and four inches off her waist over the next six months.

Example 2: Mike

Mike is forty-five years old. He was a lifelong weight lifter until he hurt his back several years ago. Since then, he has slowly gained twenty pounds. He is 5' 9" and close to 200 pounds. His waist is thirty-eight inches.

His current diet is a standard American diet. He eats three big meals a day and has become interested in the keto diet, which we decide is a great beginning structure. Mike is resistant to tracking or weighing and measuring his food and also does not like the idea of pricking his finger for the blood keto measurements. He prefers to just follow the diet and allow his results to tell him what's working.

Over the first and second weeks, we find Mike's HEC and SHMEC are in check and he is losing some fat and inches around his waist. Week three sees all of his results reverse when a cheat meal turns into a cheat week. He ends that week up overall in weight with waist measurement down. I explain to Mike that the strict approach he is taking with the keto diet is not sustainable for all people and often can lead to this type of restrict-and-binge behavior. He opts to continue on.

Over the next two weeks of Mike being consistent with the diet, we see no change in weight or inches despite HEC and SHMEC being in check. At this point, I convince Mike to start tracking his food intake and also actually measuring his ketones in his blood. He does. We find he is indeed in ketosis for brief periods of time but is also overeating substantially. Because HEC and SHMEC remain stable, we begin to cut down Mike's calories. His carbs are already low, so we begin to cut back on the avocado, cream, and nuts he is eating. We easily shave 500 calories off his diet this way.

Mike begins to see his weight and waist decline, but at this point, his HEC and SHMEC start to go out of check.

We work the five-step process, first adding lean protein (egg whites, grilled chicken, and bison) and two large salads (one with breakfast and one with dinner). This helps, but he still is feeling cravings at times. We try adding a little more fat to the diet as well as a little starch. In the end, we find that a diet with a little more fat and protein in the morning but a little more carb and less fat at night is what helps control hunger and cravings. Mike continues to lose weight and fat in a sporadic fashion. We use this to help accelerate his results, giving him two weeks on a stricter diet and two weeks on a more relaxed maintenance plan.

His dietary approach goes from keto (mostly fat) to more primal (fat and protein) to more paleo (higher protein, lower fat, and lower carbs). This approach allows him to not just lose the weight but maintain it. He ends up at a lean 180 pounds and a thirty-three-inch waist.

IT'S ALL ABOUT YOU

Becoming a metabolic detective also will require you to ditch the dieter mindset of "If I do a particular thing, I will look a certain way." If you were not born with a model's physique, you will not magically gain one by adhering to a certain diet or exercise regime. You will not become taller or smaller boned with more interesting features. You cannot alter your genetics. If you are pear shaped, you will become a more toned, less pronounced pear shape. However, most people believe if they start running, they're eventually going to look like an elite marathon runner. They don't understand that a marathon runner has a particular genetic propensity that makes them look that way. More often than not, people don't look the way they look because of what they're doing; they're doing what they're doing because of the way they look.

I'm a perfect example of this. The first sport I ever played as a child was soccer. I can remember running around the field, back and forth, again and again, and absolutely hating every single second of it.

I've always been big and muscular, even as a kid, so that particular sport did exactly nothing for me. When my father asked me at the end of the season if I wanted to sign up for the following year, my answer was a swift "*No.*" The next year, I went out for football. Now I was home. The "start, stop, go hard, stop, sprint, stop" of it all spoke perfectly to my physicality. It was the first time I realized there truly is no escaping our genetic propensity.

There's also no escaping the things we love. We can't help what we like and don't like, but in some cases, what we like isn't doing us any favors. For example, if you're someone who loves running, you have to understand that although it might be psychologically beneficial for you, it might not be physiologically effective for fat loss. Running might be like your therapy, a time when your mind can rest and you can enjoy all those endorphins. But if you're not challenging your body to do more than the leisurely job it's become accustomed to, your body will not reap the same level of reward. On the other hand, running too much could lead you to eat more than you normally would. You have to be aware enough to know when something isn't contributing to both your psychological and physical goals and change things up to make sure you're getting the maximum benefits.

That being said, don't force yourself to do a particular exercise just because you think you have to for whatever reason. I know a woman in her thirties who had a huge growth spurt around age thirteen and shot up to 5' 9". By the time she got to high school, everyone just assumed she'd play basketball because of her height, including the school's coach. At their urging, she tried out and made the team but quickly learned it was not at all the sport for her. She's naturally passive, so the aggression the sport required of her launched her outside her comfort zone to the point where she was in tears after almost every game. But she stuck with it because she thought she had to. In the off-season, she joined the track team to stay in shape for basketball. There, she discovered she absolutely loved distance running.

She wasn't the star of the team, but she looked forward to every practice and every meet. After three seasons, she quit the basketball team and has never picked up a ball since. She does, however, still run at least ten miles every week and regularly competes in races all over her city.

The same principle holds true with food. If you love chocolate, you can't pretend like you're never going to have it again. You need to find a way to have chocolate. Maybe you allow yourself a designated small amount or find a low-calorie cocoa drink you like. Part of being a metabolic detective is understanding there is going to be a give and take between the things you love and the things that are going to benefit you most. You won't get to do exactly what you want to do all day every day, but you can design a lifestyle you can love and live with long term.

If you started out as a more intuitive eater, it might be time to become disciplined about documenting your meals and calorie counting. If you're a lifelong calorie counter, it's likely time to train yourself to become more intuitive about eating. Remember the scenario where HEC and SHMEC were in check but you weren't losing fat? That may require a stricter calorie-counting approach to fix. When HEC and SHMEC are out of check, you may need a more intuitive approach, manipulating meals until you land on the right strategy.

Figuring out the right approach for you can take some work, but the more you understand how all the parts of the puzzle are working together, the better choices you can make.

SUCCESSFUL WEIGHT
LOSS MAINTAINERS

At this point, you might be feeling a little overwhelmed. You might even be frustrated and convinced when it comes to metabolism and weight loss, it is impossible for you to make any lasting change. But I want to assure you there are many, many people who have lost weight and kept it off for years.

In fact, researchers at the National Weight Control Registry have been tracking successful weight loss maintainers for years. Even though these individuals are in the minority, they most definitely exist and they have important lessons to teach.

Although I know I've been encouraging you to stick with what works best for you, the truth is, most of these individuals do weigh and measure. Not only do they have a way to track their food and calories, but they are also meticulous about tracking changes in their body. I can't tell you how many times I have had patients tell me, "No matter what I do, I simply can't lose weight." Then when I ask them if they have ever weighed, tracked, and measured their food calories and macros, they say no. This is a lot like giving a beginning piano student Beethoven's most complex piano concerto and expecting them to be able to play any of it.

TRACKING AND WEIGHT LOSS

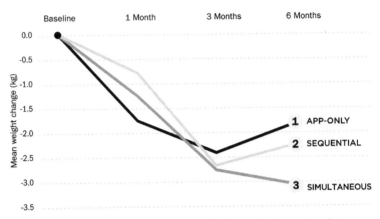

Comparing Self-Monitoring Strategies for Weight Loss in a Smartphone App: Randomized Controlled Trial. JMIR mHealth and uHealth, 2019; 7 (2) PMID: 30816851

STUDY OVERVIEW:

105 subjects between the ages of 21 and 65 were divided into three different groups.

3 GROUPS:

1 Track food for 3 months.

2 Track weight 1 month, then add in food tracking for 2 months. Habit and nutrition education as well.

3 A combination of groups 1 and 2 (tracking weight and food, and education for three months).

· Minor differences in weight lost.

· **Tracking food may be the most important component of weight loss.**

· App used was *myfitnesspal.*

STUDY RESULTS:

· Group 1 (tracking food only) lost 5 pounds.

· Group 2 (tracking weight first, then adding food tracking later, plus nutrition and habit education) lost 6 pounds.

· Group 3 (tracking weight and food from the start along with coaching on habits, goal setting, and nutrition) lost 6 pounds.

· Group 3 continued to lose weight after the trial, while groups 1 and 2 regained a small amount.

· Those most diligent with tracking food lost the most weight.

The metabolism does not care about your convenience concerns. It is unfazed by your annoyance and it could care less if any of this is frustrating for you. If you want results that last, there simply are certain things you must learn, practice, and master. Each individual has to find a way to consistently, accurately, and continuously monitor their food intake.

Not only do successful weight loss maintainers obsess over what they eat, but they also are hyperfocused on how much they weigh. In fact, they monitor their bodies daily. They take weight, body composition, or circumference measurements more frequently than unsuccessful dieters. Research has actually shown that those who monitor their physical appearance and attributes daily fare better than those who monitor it only weekly or less.[24] Again, this does not need to be weight. It could be any measurements you want to take, as long as you take them often.

One of the benefits of frequently weighing and measuring food and body weight is the lessons you learn. Each fluctuation is feedback and a lesson. Perhaps you'll see how every time you have wine, you seem to weigh more over the next several days.

Maybe you'll start to realize that the two tablespoons of peanut butter you use to curb cravings is actually more like five when you actually weigh it out, adding hundreds of calories to your daily intake. Perhaps you notice that days after exercise, you are a little heavier and hold a little bit of water. All of this offers valuable learning and teaches you what is important and meaningful to pay attention to and what is not. The more data points, the better.

Successful individuals also are consistent about movement. None of them are sitters. What these weight loss maintainers tell us is that you will not and cannot be successful long term if you are not going to move. These individuals move constantly and consistently. Both movement and metabolics are part of their daily routines, but movement is most critical, and in most cases, that means walking.

Need more convincing? Here is an overview of stats taken directly from the National Weight Control Registry's summary of findings:[25]

- The registry is 80 percent female (average age forty-five, average weight 145) and 20 percent male (average age forty-nine, average weight 190).
- The average weight lost by registry participants is 66 pounds (ranging from 30 to 300).
- The average duration of weight loss maintenance is five years (ranging from one year to sixty-six years).
- Some of the participants lost the weight fast (over months) and some slowly (over years).
- The amount of people who lost the weight on their own is about equal to those who used some type of diet system or program.
- Ninety-eight percent modified their food intake in some way.
- Ninety-four percent increased their physical activity, with walking being by far the most common.
- Most all continue to monitor food and physical activity.
- Seventy-eight percent eat breakfast.
- Seventy-five percent weigh themselves frequently.
- Sixty-two percent watch little TV (less than ten hours per week).
- Ninety percent exercise (about one hour per day on average).

This research shows that even though losing weight is hard, keeping it off is even harder. Luckily, we have good data that tells us the behaviors that are most important.

The most important thing to remember is that the change required to lose fat and maintain a fit, healthy, lean metabolism must be a permanent one. This is why through this book I have focused on giving you the requisite knowledge to understand how to construct your own fat loss lifestyle—a system built for you by you and a lifestyle you can own, love, and live with long term.

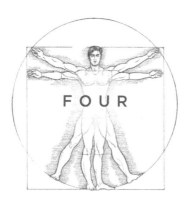

FOUR

THE METABOLIC ARCHITECT

B y now, you know that if your approach to nutrition lacks balance between calorie counting and intuitive eating, you're missing most of the messages your metabolism is sending you. When you're only counting calories, you're ignoring the needs of your hormones. If you're only eating intuitively and letting your biofeedback from hormones call all the shots, you could be overeating (or undereating) and thereby throwing your metabolism into a stress spiral without even knowing it. In either scenario, you're only fighting half the battle. Don't let yourself feel too defeated—most people start out right where you are. But in order to master your metabolism and use it to your best advantage, you have to pay attention to both calories and hormones.

Remember the law of individuality from Chapter One? It states that each one of us has different physiology, psychology, personal preferences, and practical circumstances, all of which contribute to how we think about diet and exercise. For some people, counting, weighing, and measuring everything they eat and drink seems like an absurd idea because they are either crazy busy, constantly traveling, or dealing with any of the countless other uncertainties life can throw at us. Some people simply hate the idea of it. Others might love all the math that goes into tracking every calorie or might just find it to be the most helpful way to learn about their good and bad habits. Others might trust their own intuition when it comes to food and see no point in keeping track of every little thing. All of this is fine—each person's relationship with their own well-being is very much an individual thing. However—and this is the big *however* that most people would prefer to ignore—it's important to realize that the approach you prefer is *not always the approach that works best.*

Just because you naturally gravitate toward something does not mean it's enough. Again, if you're doing everything right and not getting results, you're not doing everything right.

You have to let data and results drive your actions, and that means you might need a different approach despite your natural proclivities. If you're taking an intuitive approach and it's not working, you have to challenge yourself to become more intentional about paying attention to what you're consuming. If you can't function without a food scale and meal plan, you have to take a step back and learn to understand it's not only about the things you eat; it's about how they impact your HEC and SCHMEC. Again, neither of these approaches is bad, but if they're not working on their own, it's time to reevaluate your actions.

Altering habits can be challenging because bias and dogma play big roles in how we think about nutrition. We tend to let ourselves become entrenched in believing there's one right thing we know to be true, and anything else is nonsense. But when we do that, we've resigned ourselves to never getting results. Bias and dogma are the parents of ignorance and arrogance—when your beliefs blind you from seeing any other way of doing something, you are bound for failure. I know this from experience as I am living proof of the problems you can cause for yourself when you become too married to your own way of doing things.

When I was in my early twenties and in medical school, I was a strict vegetarian. Mind you, this was during my ignorant, arrogant, young male days, which I will use as an excuse for why I was all about pushing this diet on anyone who would listen to me. I started researching some of the science around it because I wanted more ammo for my argument. Yet, what I ended up learning was the opposite of what I was hoping to find, and I ended up proving myself wrong. At the time, I had recently started experiencing some health difficulties and eventually was diagnosed with hypothyroidism, among other things. I believe that diagnosis was a direct result of how dogmatic I had been about adhering to a vegetarian lifestyle. This is not to say vegetarianism is bad—it can be great for a lot of people—but it wasn't a lifestyle that worked well with my own unique physiology.

It was a hard lesson to learn, albeit an important one. Being too narrow and rigid in my beliefs had gotten me into some serious trouble, but the experience taught me that if you're really serious about your health and well-being, you have to rely on the data and use all the tools available to you. Good metabolic detectives don't ignore anything. By focusing only on calories, you're ignoring HEC and SCHMEC and treating metabolism like a calculator. When you rely only on intuition, you're only listening to biofeedback. As you know by now, metabolism is a barometer, and to understand how to work with its adaptable nature, you have to be able to switch back and forth between the two.

QUANTITY AND QUALITY

People often like to say that quality always matters more than quantity. But when it comes to metabolism, both matter equally. **Quantity** pertains to calories, or how much fuel you're taking in. **Quality** pertains to hormones, or the types of foods you're eating and how they're impacting HEC and SHMEC. To achieve successful and sustainable fat loss, you have to be paying attention to both. There is no way around it—you *must* have both a calorie deficit *and* a sustained calorie deficit (i.e., hormonal metabolic balance).

Believing that all you have to do is "eat healthily" or "eat clean" is a regimented, prescribed dieter's tactic, and we both know you're better than that. Even if you think you're making the best choices possible, it is entirely feasible (and easy) for absolutely anyone to overeat the right foods. You need to focus on quantity to make sure that doesn't happen, and the more you do that, the easier it becomes. Over time, your understanding of quantity will begin to inform your thinking around quality.

For instance, I have logged thousands of hours of counting, weighing, and measuring food.

By now, all I have to do is look at a typical Chipotle bowl full of rice, chicken, beans, salsa, and cheese, and I can tell you roughly how many calories are in it. I know what eight ounces of chicken looks like. I know what a cup of black beans looks like. I know what a cup of rice looks like. I can look at all of those things together and just know how many calories are in the bowl.

Most people think good intuition is some kind of magical quality only a select few possess. It's not. As mentioned in the previous chapter, intuition is the integration of all your senses plus experience (remember Sully landing on the Hudson?). You can fine-tune your intuition around food by learning as much as you can about what you put into your body. Do you know what a protein is? A starch? A carbohydrate? Some of what you learn might surprise you. It might be a shock to discover that Starbucks Frappuccino you get every morning actually has around 800 calories. You might scoff at how small one recommended serving of whole-grain cereal really looks. It all starts with awareness, and once you add in the measuring, your intuition will continue to sharpen.

ENERGY OUT

Although it's important to track the fuel you take in each day, it also helps to know how your energy is being expended. You burn calories twenty-four hours a day, not only when you actively, intentionally exercise.

Of course, you expend energy when you exercise, which is known as exercise-associated thermogenesis or EAT. Going about your daily life also burns calories; non-exercise activity thermo-genesis (NEAT) refers to the amount of energy you burn by walk-ing around, doing chores, working at your desk, chasing after the kids—just living, basically. Our bodies use energy during diges-tion, too. The thermic effect of food, or TEF, relates to the amount of energy you burn when you chew, break down, and take energy from food.

You also burn calories when you sleep or lie around. Resting energy expenditure (REE), also known as basal metabolic rate (BMR), measures the calories you burn even when you're not doing anything. If you only stayed in bed flat on your back and did nothing all day long, you would still burn a certain number of calories through the energy expended to perform bodily func-tions like breathing and maintaining your heartbeat. You cal-culate your REE or BMR partly based on your muscle mass. But don't get too excited—you can't just put on a pound of muscle and have your REE go through the roof. It only goes up by an estimated six to thirty calories max per pound of muscle you put on your body. A pound of fat uses three to six calories per pound. This tells you that any extra muscle you gain only has a big advan-tage when it is moving, not when it is sitting still.

To determine how your body expends energy and how many calories are burned, all four aspects of metabolism—EAT, NEAT, TEF, and REE—have to be calculated. This might seem like com-mon sense, but most people make incorrect assumptions about each of these factors. For example, EAT accounts for only about 5 percent of extra calories burned, whereas NEAT accounts for nearly 15 percent. This illustrates the difference between moving and exercising. As far as calorie use goes, you are far better off moving all day and not exercising than you are sitting all day and then doing a sixty-minute HIIT class. This illustrates why movement is given an entire category in the 4Ms.

CALORIE-COUNTING SHORTCUTS

Calculating your baseline calorie level is easy: simply take your body weight in pounds and multiply it by ten. This is a crude estimate of calorie needs but can act as a good starting rule of thumb for what may be required to begin seeing fat loss. If you're an athlete or more performance-oriented, multiply by fifteen. If your goal is to put on muscle, multiply by twenty. These are good general guidelines for most people. But remember, your metabolism is unique.

Your job is to always follow the structured flexibility approach. These gross calculations are just another form of structure; it's up to you to pay attention to whether they generate the results you want, and you will need to be flexible in your adjustments.

Regardless of what kind of person you are, you must always remember your metabolism does not care what you think about calories. Some people believe if they go below 1,000 calories, their body will shut down. That's not true. If your BMR is 2,000 and you take in only 1,000 calories, those extra calories are going to come from the fat stored in your body. Only HEC and SHMEC can tell you when you've gone too low with calorie intake.

Tracking all of this can help you better understand why you might not be seeing your weight loss goals come to fruition. Let's say through all of this, your burn 2,500 a day. If you're eating 2,600 calories, you're never going to lose weight. It's simple math, and there is an array of total daily energy expenditure (TDEE) calculators out there that can help you figure it all out. TDEE is a measurement of all the parts of metabolism we just mentioned (REE, NEAT, EAT, TEF). TDEE simply adds the activity factor. It is a more accurate way of determining caloric needs; however, it too can never be exact. The metabolism is adjusting calorie needs constantly. It is a living, breathing system, and it is wrong to think there is an exact calorie number you need. Even if your metabolic rate has been tested under laboratory conditions, that number is not exact. Calorie calculations are always best guesses, and in the end, they will be proven accurate only if they deliver results.

This is never going to be an exact science because, as you know by now, your metabolism is always adapting and changing. If your metabolism feels like too much energy is going out, it is capable of making you less motivated to exercise. It might make you stop fidgeting or moving in your sleep. It can decrease its resting energy expenditure (BMR) by adjusting the thyroid hormone. It can work to constrain the number of calories you burn in other areas as a result of your typical exercise session. The only true way to know if you are in a calorie deficit is achieving weight loss.

Your metabolism has many different ways of compensating, and because of these fluctuations, there is no one formula that will tell you the exact quantity of calories you're burning on any given day. But even having a general idea will help you make decisions that will lead to sustainable success as it will give you something to compare to what you're actually taking in.

Furthermore, although calorie counting can give you a wider view of what's happening with your body, it has nothing to do with shutting down hunger and cravings or improving mood and sleep. You have to be paying attention to exactly what you're taking into your body and how it impacts you, and this is where quality comes in. If you only focus on creating a calorie deficit, you risk throwing hormonal balance off.

For example, I have a friend who is an ex-bodybuilder. He is 5' 8" and 190 pounds. He has no health issues. I'm 5' 10", 225 pounds, and I have a thyroid issue. Even if we both expend the same amount of energy a day, my friend can eat about 4,000 calories per day and maintain his weight, whereas if I go above 2,500 calories, I start gaining weight. I have to think about my TDEE in the context of my thyroid condition. I learned this by running these equations and paying attention to how my metabolism was reacting to different scenarios. Even though the numbers might be far off for me, I never would have learned how to adjust the quality of what I was taking in without knowing them. Quality and quantity must be attended to equally. This is a perfect example of how having a calorie deficit *and* hormonal balance are both essential to creating the best diet for your unique physiology.

QUALITY CONTROL

One of the best ways to achieve hormonal balance is by understanding what macronutrients do. Macronutrients are the things your body needs most—protein, carbohydrates, and fat (some like to think of water, fiber, and alcohol as their own macro categories as well).

For most people, protein, fiber, and water are the best way to shut down hunger, but everyone has an individual response to macronutrients. You might have to play around with them a bit to find what works best for you. For example, chicken and broccoli is a very low-calorie, hunger-suppressing meal. Leaving the skin on the chicken will add calories to be sure, but you also might find that it impacts how well that particular meal keeps your hunger at bay—does it keep you satiated longer, or does that addition of fat amp up cravings later in the day?

Another way to figure out how fat impacts you is to swap the eggs in your usual morning veggies omelet with egg whites. You're not taking out the yolks because they're "bad" for you—in fact, yolks are one of the most power-packed, nutrient-rich foods you can find. But for your purposes, starting with protein, fiber, and water first will help you see how bringing in other macronutrients like fat and starch affects you. You can always add the yolks back in later or mix in a small amount of feta cheese to make the omelet tastier. Or you might find it more beneficial to add some more egg whites plus some extra water-based vegetables. That combination might suppress your hunger even more, and you may not even be able to finish the whole thing. Then you can start reintroducing yolks back or using butter when you cook the eggs, paying attention to any changes in HEC and SHMEC all along the way.

This process should help you see that you're not just eating the egg white veggie omelet because it's considered healthy—you're eating it because it's loaded with protein, fiber, and water, and it offers the dual benefit of calorie reduction and hormone balance, the combination you should always be striving for.

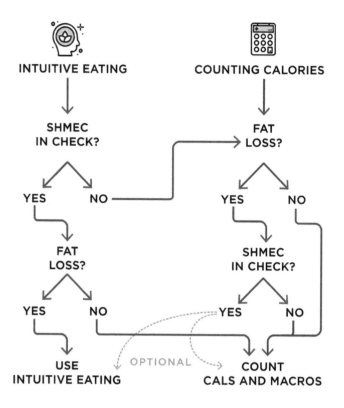

PROTEIN TRACKING

One of the most well-studied and effective methods of eating comes from understanding protein. If you were to ask me, "Jade, what is the one thing you have seen be more effective than anything else in attaining and maintaining weight loss?" I would likely go back and forth between three things: walking, weight training, and protein intake. Walking helps lower stress hormones and sensitizes the body to insulin. In this way, it can be a powerful control mechanism for keeping hunger and cravings in check. Weight training helps make sure that the body loses less muscle during weight loss and therefore works to mitigate metabolic compensation and weight gain rebound. Protein does all of these things. It helps control hunger, balance cravings, *and* maintain muscle mass.

If you were to substitute equal protein calories in place of carbohydrate or fat calories, you would almost certainly lose weight and most of that weight would be fat. Eating more protein causes you to eat less naturally. In this way, it creates an "accidental" calorie deficit. Protein also acts as a signal to maintain muscle mass rather than lose it. Protein is the most thermogenic of the macronutrients. This means it takes more energy to digest, absorb, and assimilate protein. It is also the most satiating macronutrient. This means it fills you up fast and keeps you full and without cravings for long periods of time.

The science on the weight loss and health benefits of protein intake is now crystal clear in the research. Not only does a higher protein diet *not* cause issues, but it is also now known to be exceedingly healthy. This is true even at levels over one gram per pound of body weight. The diagram below demonstrates the amounts of protein you should be shooting for based on the existing body of literature.

You can use this understanding about protein to make things much easier to track and manage. One of the most successful tools I have ever used in clinical practice is to just count grams of protein and nothing else. I tell my clients to get at least their lean body weight in grams of protein daily and as much as their body weight in grams of protein. Lean body mass is your body weight in pounds subtracted by your body fat in pounds. Lean body mass is how much muscle, water, and organ tissue you have. If you think in kilograms, you'll want to convert that number to pounds to use this tool. So break out your mobile device and do the conversion.

HOW MUCH PROTEIN PER DAY?

	MAINTAIN	FAT LOSS	MUSCLE GAIN
NORMAL-WEIGHT SEDENTARY	0.54–0.82 g/lbs 1.2–1.8 g/kg	0.54–0.68 g/lbs 1.2–1.5 g/kg	N/A
OVERWEIGHT SEDENTARY	N/A	0.54–0.68 g/lbs 1.2–1.5 g/kg	N/A
ACTIVE OR ATHLETE	0.6–1.00 g/lbs 1.4–2.2 g/kg	1.2–1.5g/lbs 2.2–3.3 g/kg	0.6–1.5g/lbs 1.4–3.3 g/kg
PREGNANT	0.75–0.80g/lbs 1.66–1.77 g/kg	N/A	N/A

References/Sources:

PMID: 24092765   PMID: 22215165   PMID: 25733478
PMID: 28630601   PMID: 19841581   www.examine.com
PMID: 26500462   PMID: 29497353   www.consumerlab.com
PMID: 25527661   PMID: 22510792

This method is so powerful because it allows you to focus on only one thing—getting your protein grams in. Surprisingly, when most people do this, they find a few things. First, they discover they are usually too full to even eat all that protein. They also find they eat less of everything else. This protein focus method is about as close to magic as exists in the weight loss world. If you are extremely overweight, you can stick to the lean body mass number. I have found that very few people, with the exceptions of athletes and weightlifters, are able to consume over 200 g of protein even if they try. I often make 200 g of protein the ceiling for most inactive overweight individuals. Later, toward the end of this book when we talk about maintenance, you'll see me mention this strategy again in regard to the concept of "nutritional keystones." This little protein trick may be the most powerful "hack" in this entire book.

ARE YOU SATISFIED?

Quality and quantity can handle hunger, but what about satisfaction?

Relieving the hunger you feel in your gut does not necessarily result in quenching your brain's desire for a certain taste or texture. Satiation is about hunger; satisfaction is about cravings. Satisfaction is linked to those cravings you feel in your head, and you don't have to ignore them. You really can eat whatever you want, as long as you continue to watch how much you eat and pay attention to the effect it has on your biofeedback. Every person has to find a way to make food enjoyable while keeping calories reasonable and HEC and SHMEC in check. You can't eat only chicken and broccoli forever. That's the MO of an uneducated dieter who's only relying on what they think they know to be true. You also can't eat whatever you want and think just because you're counting up all those calories, everything will be fine. You have to be able to do both.

As you're making your food choices, it helps to think about what each option is offering. For instance, if you were given either five chicken breasts or five doughnuts to eat in an entire day, which will you be able to finish, and which will leave you with leftovers? Most people can eat five doughnuts throughout the course of a day with no problem (heck, some people can do that before lunch). Almost no one is going to be able to eat five chicken breasts. Yet, one boneless skinless chicken breast has roughly the same number of calories as one doughnut—250 or so. So what makes them different?

It all comes down to the macronutrient ratio, especially the protein. The protein in the chicken is highly satiating. It suppresses the appetite. The chicken breast is also very low in fat and has no carbohydrates. The doughnut, however, is exactly the opposite. The doughnut has virtually no protein. It is loaded with fat and sugar, giving it less satiating potential. That means there is no logic in grabbing a doughnut and expecting it to quash your hunger. In fact, foods rich in the combinations of fat, sugar, and salt, like a doughnut, have been shown to trigger more cravings for similar highly palatable foods. Although this is not true for all people, it is a good bet that it is true for most.

You might grab a doughnut because it tastes good and satisfies a craving, but don't be surprised if your stomach is rumbling within the hour and you find yourself reaching for another one. The chicken breast, however, is far more likely to hold you until your next meal, no snacking needed.

This is the way you want to start thinking about food. It is not just about what that food does to you in the moment. You also should be thinking, "If I eat this food, will it help me eat less and better-quality foods later? Or will I be likely to eat more and worse foods later?" Food is not simply a bunch of calories; it is also a packet of information for your metabolism.

GETTING STARTED

Although I am not a proponent of a one-size-fits-all diet, there is a way of eating that offers a perfectly synergistic merging of quality and quantity: the Five S diet. That stands for soups, salads, scrambles, shakes, and stir-fries, though in my mind, those are all really the same thing. Soups are essentially wet salads; scrambles are salads with eggs; shakes are blended salads; and stir-fries are hot salads. Skillet meals also count as stir-fries. The idea is to eat mainly low-carb, low-fat, low-starch versions of each of these because those are the things that will help you get calories down and hormones under control. Once that happens, you can start to add some starch, fat, sugar, salt, and alcohol to make your meals more enjoyable.

Ideally, you want 90 percent of what you eat to be the Five Ss, 10 percent to be starch, sugar, fat, salt, and alcohol, and 1 percent to be junk food. Although this is a fairly intuitive way of eating, you can't stop paying attention to calories. Remember, even though it would be far less likely compared to other foods, you can still overeat all of these things.

The Five S diet is a more intuitive approach than the counting, weighing, and measuring approach. If you'd prefer to have even more flexibility, you can use the hand-measuring approach, which is even more intuitive.

This is based on the idea that at each meal, you should have two palms' worth of vegetables, one palm's worth of protein, half a palm of starch, and a thumb of fat. You also could use the plate method: half the plate should be vegetables, a quarter should be protein, and a quarter should be high-fiber starch and/or fat.

Each of these approaches will work differently for each person, and there is no magic in any of them. Every one is just a different way to provide a beginning structure. As is the case with all things pertaining to metabolism, it's up to you to determine what works best for you and be flexible in your approach in creating the perfect diet for you.

THE "5S DIET"

Eat 90 percent or more of your food in the form of low-fat, low-carb versions of these items. There is nothing wrong with fat or carbs, but they provide less hunger suppression and more calories compared to these water, fiber, and protein-rich options.

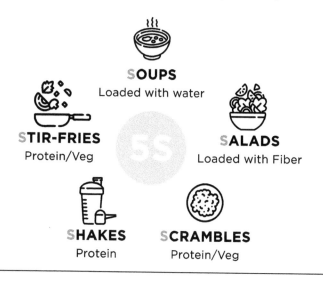

SOUPS
Loaded with water

STIR-FRIES
Protein/Veg

SALADS
Loaded with Fiber

SHAKES
Protein

SCRAMBLES
Protein/Veg

- Eat less fat, starch, and salt
- Eat enough to make your meals enjoyable
- Eat to your tolerance
- Be careful with combining these elements as it could trigger overeating and future cravings

- Reduce sugar
- Reduce alcohol
- Use only occasionally
- Use if buffer food
- Avoid completely if trigger food

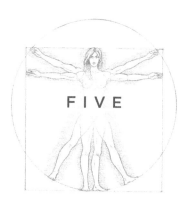

FIVE

THE METABOLIC ENGINEER

S ee if this sounds familiar: You decide it's finally time to drop those last ten pounds, so you start a new low-calorie diet and begin exercising harder than you ever have. You're really motivated for the first few weeks, and you start to see some minor results. Then things plateau, you get frustrated and fed up, and before you know it, you're back to snacking around the clock and vegging on the couch. After a few weeks of that, your pants don't fit anymore, and it's back to dieting and exercising. Soon enough, your battery is completely drained again, and out come the ice cream and Pringles.

Have you ever found yourself caught in this vicious cycle? Most people have. It's extremely common to bounce back and forth between being a dieter and a couch potato over and over and over, never seeing any real change in your body or watching the weight pile on as those stints on the couch get longer and longer. In this case, the very thing dieters are trying to do to lose weight is also the thing causing them to regain the weight. In other words, the eat less, exercise more (ELEM) approach *almost always* leads to eat more, exercise less (EMEL).

So who is putting more stress on the metabolism: the dieter or the couch potato? Unfortunately, it's a tie.

Remember that metabolism is a stress barometer, and one of the sources of stress it's always measuring is calorie intake versus output. If that gap gets too wide in either direction, the metabolism runs into problems. The couch potato has too much intake, not enough output; the dieter has too much output, not enough intake. Think of your body like an apartment. If there's nothing in it, you can't function. But if you're a hoarder and you fill your apartment up with way too much stuff, you also can't live in it properly.

The dieter is the extreme minimalist; the couch potato is the hoarder. Both will throw HEC and SHMEC out of check and all but guarantee you'll never see real lasting weight loss. You need something in between that makes life more livable.

METABOLIC TOGGLES

You have to find a way to close the calorie gap and convince the metabolism it does not need to be stressed out, and there are specific ways you can do this. By understanding the four metabolic toggles you can use to increase or decrease stress on your metabolism, you can determine what state will best help you achieve your goals.

THE METABOLIC TOGGLES

- The metabolism is an adaptive system. It responds better to change and challenge.
- Doing nothing but the "eat less, exercise more" model can work against results.
- Cycling between the 4 metabolic toggles may reduce metabolic adaptation.
- There are many approaches to cycling (seasonal, menstrual, daily, weekly).
- ESES (eat some, exercise some) is maintenance (an isocaloric state).

ELEM	EMEM
EAT LESS, EXERCISE MORE	EAT MORE, EXERCISE MORE
DIETER	**ATHLETE**
Limit to 2–4 weeks max	Works great in 3-month training blocks
Early spring	Late spring to early fall

ESES

HUNTER-GATHERER	COUCH POTATO
Best toggle for year-round living	Limit to 4–7 days
Keto and fasting fit well here	Good after intense training blocks
Winter	Late fall

ELEL	EMEL
EAT LESS, EXERCISE LESS	EAT MORE, EXERCISE LESS

* Sleep, Hunger, Mood, Energy, Cravings (SHMEC) can guide you. When SHMEC goes out of check, it is a good indication it's time to switch to another toggle.

Eat Less, Exercise More

To the typical dieter who is using the ELEM approach, everything looks like calories. The only thing they are concerned about is cutting out as much of those calories as possible, either by practically starving themselves or by totally overdoing their workouts.

They are in no way paying attention to the language their metabolism is speaking. Instead, they are trying to force their own will on metabolism, which we know by now is completely pointless. They believe all they need is willpower, and failure is only for the weak-minded.

These are the same people who wake up on the first warm day of spring and head out for their first run of the year, convinced they're going to instantly burn off all the fat they've been carrying around all winter. Inevitably, they end up hurting themselves and land right back on the very couch they had to peel themselves off. But don't worry, they'll try again. And again. *And again.* In fact, they'll continue to ping-pong back and forth between being a dieter and a couch potato indefinitely until they wake up and realize their metabolism is really the one running the show.

The dieter thinks of willpower as a fully charged cell phone—they have a full battery, so they believe they can keep going forever. But they forget that eventually, that battery is going to drain and they will have to recharge it. After so long, they find themselves with no power left, and suddenly, that couch is looking like a great spot to hang out while they wait for the battery to power back up.

Rarely is ELEM effective. Most often, it leads to failure and does nothing but convince your metabolism it's starving, which makes it compensate and therefore undo any of the hard work you think you're doing. If, for some reason, you feel the need to try this toggle, do not do it for much longer than two weeks and definitely not more than four. If you do, you may end up doing more harm than good.

The good news is that when you use the ELEM toggle sparingly for short periods with long breaks in between, it starts working the way we all think it should. There is nothing inherently bad about ELEM—it's just overused. Think about it: your metabolism is an adaptive system. If you try to do the same thing day in and day out over and over again, the metabolism will adapt and conserve. By now, you know how to spot this. The metabolism is always talking to you, and when HEC and SHMEC go out of check, you can be sure the ELEM toggle is no longer going to be effective. Likewise, if your weight loss results slow or plateau, you know you have engaged this toggle for too long, and it is time to give it a break.

The ELEM toggle has you pulling on the metabolism from both sides. You are creating calorie deficits through food and exercise. That large gap in intake and output is what causes the metabolism to become more rigid and stingy in its fat usage. By giving yourself breaks from this metabolic toggle and using it intelligently and sparingly, you will be able to benefit from it once again.

Eat More, Exercise Less

EMEL is the couch potato toggle. It is the opposite of ELEM. It too generates a large calorie gap, but it just does so in the opposite direction. Isn't it interesting that the undereating, overexercising dieter and the overconsuming, underexercising couch potato both have issues with HEC and SHMEC? That is because both of these toggles, when done for extended periods of time, cause a rigid dysfunctional metabolic state.

That being said, the couch potato toggle does have some utility and should not be abandoned altogether. When very short-lived, it can provide some benefit toward recovery from training. It also can provide a much-needed break from ELEM. For athletes and those wanting to gain muscle, it can be a useful toggle to employ.

EAT LESS, EXERCISE MORE PROTOCOL

Calculating Calories and Macronutrients (macros)

- Set grams of protein equal to lean body weight in pounds.
- Suggested starting macro percent is 30:40:30 (carbs, protein, fat).
- Calculate calories based on protein level (see examples).
- Walk 10–20K steps daily, and exercise 4–7 days per week.
- Adjust calories and macros based on results and biofeedback.

Remember!
4 cal per gram of carbohydrate,
4 cal per gram of protein, 9 cal per gram of fat

185-Pound Female, 30% Fat

Set protein to 185 − (185 × 0.30) = 130g

130 × 4 cal = 520 cal protein

520 ÷ 0.40 = 1300 total cal

(1300 × 0.30 carbs) ÷ 4 cal = 98g carb

(1300 × .30 fat) ÷ 9 cal = 43g fat

1300 total cal
98g carb, 130g protein, 43g fat

240-Pound Male, 27% Fat

Set protein to 240 − (240 × 0.27) =175g

175 × 4 cal =700 cal protein

700 ÷ 0.40 = 1750 total cal

(1750 × 0.30 carbs) ÷ 4 cal = 131g carb

(1750 × 0.30 fat) ÷ 9 cal = 58g fat

1750 total cal
131g carb, 175g protein, 58g fat

Just like eating less can slow metabolic rate, eating more can elevate it. This has led many coaches to use refeeds (a period of time, usually a few days, of eating slightly more than normal) and cheat meals with their clients to get their metabolism moving again. This approach can work, but it also has tremendous potential to backfire. Although eating more can raise metabolic rate, it typically does not do so to the same degree that dieting lowers it. Also, eating more usually means eating large amounts of highly palatable foods rich in the combination of fat, sugar, starch, salt, and/or alcohol. Think burgers, pizza, pastries, and pasta. These foods can cause more cravings for the same types of foods later. This is why cheat meals often turn into cheat months and why a refeed can turn into a feeding frenzy.

Again, you know it's not going to do much for you in the long run, so if you are a person who's trying to lose weight or maintain a loss, this is a toggle you will use sparingly. Think of a brief four-day vacation or the occasional day on the weekend or a recovery day from extreme sport or exercise the day prior. The max amount of time you should spend in this toggle is four days and definitely not longer than seven. Anything more is likely to start working against you.

Eat Less, Exercise Less

ELEL is the hunter-gatherer toggle. Think back to the early days of man. People were nomadic and only ate what they foraged. They moved all day every day. No, they weren't swinging kettlebells or running marathons—they simply were moving from place to place. Their NEAT was hugely elevated, and they ate relatively sparingly. Food wasn't readily available, and highly palatable, calorie-dense foods were scarce. People were hard-pressed to take in a predictable number of calories from day to day, and because of the unpredictability of their environments, they created calorie deficits through food mostly, not exercise.

All the walking they did sensitized the body to insulin and reduced cortisol levels. The lower calorie state forced the body to use up its fuel reserves, meaning fat. But because the body doesn't want to start using up all of its reserves of other things like protein and amino acids, it becomes naturally motivated to move in order to find food. This is why hunter-gatherers are relatively lean. They're not super muscular, because they're not exercising a lot, but they are slender.

In today's world, the best example of a hunter-gatherer is the seventy-year-old woman you will inevitably see walking around the city if you ever go to Paris. She's holding bags of groceries full of fresh fruits and vegetables she picked up from all the markets she visited that morning. When she gets to her building, she walks up three flights of stairs to get to her fourth-floor apartment. She's very thin and healthy but not overly muscular. She's not thinking about exercise. She's just living her life the way she knows how to live it, and her lithe frame reflects that.

Parisians living the more traditional European lifestyle eat pretty much whatever they want—they just eat small amounts. They wake up and have coffee and a pastry. They have a small baguette sandwich for lunch, or perhaps some cheese and meat with a little bit of wine. Then they have a sensible dinner.

They don't deprive themselves of rich, delicious foods (which would be a true travesty in Paris), but they know that just a little is enough. You can live in ELEL indefinitely as long as HEC and SHMEC stay in check.

ELEL Macronutrient Ratio

There are several ways to calculate the calories and macronutrients for an ELEL metabolic state. You can set the calories exactly as you might with an ELEM approach: multiplying 10 by your body weight. You can then use a macronutrient ratio of 30-40-30 of carbohydrates, protein, and fat, respectively. Why this particular ratio? It most resembles the hunter-gatherer macronutrient ratio and is typically what you will get when you focus on low-fat, low-carb, high-fiber, and high-protein soups, salads, scrambles, shakes, and stir-fries.

An even better approach would be to calculate the ELEL state prioritizing the most satiating macronutrient, protein. ELEL naturally produces a low-calorie intake. Anytime calories are lower, it can trigger hunger and cravings. ELEL reduces this risk by decreasing exercise, a known stimulator of hunger. Unlike ELEM, ELEL achieves calorie deficits through decreased food alone; it does not increase exercise as well. It is wise to raise the protein intake as a proportion of total calories because protein is a powerhouse in reducing hunger. It also signals the body to not lose too much muscle. This is why we set the protein percentage to 40 percent. Higher protein with decreased exercise is a powerful one-two punch in controlling hunger and cravings.

To make this more objective, we set protein grams to the lean body mass of the individual. The lean body mass is the body weight after subtracting out fat stores and consists of muscle, bone, water, and organ tissue. You can calculate your lean body mass by understanding your body fat percentage.

- A 200-pound person with 30 percent body fat has a lean body mass of 200 minus 60, or 140. In the ELEL approach, this would be the number of protein grams consumed.

- From there, we can back-calculate the number of calories that 140 grams of protein is 40 percent of. So we multiply 140 times 4 (because there are 4 calories per gram of protein). That gives us 560 calories of protein.

- Then we cross-multiply by dividing .40 (40 percent) into 560, which gives us a total of 1,400 calories.

- From there, we calculate the fat grams by multiplying 1,400 by .30 (30 percent fat), which gives us 420 calories of fat. There are 9 calories per gram of fat, so we divide 420 by 9 to get 46.66 grams or 47 grams of fat.

- We then repeat this process with the carbs: 1,400 times .30 (30 percent carbs) again yields 420 calories. There are 4 calories per gram of carbohydrate, and 420 divided by 4 gives us 105 grams of carbohydrate.

- This leaves us with 1,400 calories with 105 grams of carbohydrate, 140 grams of protein, and 47 grams of fat.

Many will look at these numbers and question the calorie level. It is important to remember that low calories coupled with extreme or prolonged consistent exercise is very different than low calories with just walking and activities of daily living. If one were to consider the actual caloric availability of living as a hunter-gatherer, eating only what could be killed or gathered, one would realize that consistently achieving calorie intake much above 1,500 to 2,000 calories per day would be relatively difficult to do. Consider that five chicken breasts along with nearly unlimited salad greens and a few cups of berries would constitute the same type of diet calculated above and would not exceed much past 1,200 calories, despite being extremely nutritious and hunger suppressing.

EAT LESS, EXERCISE LESS PROTOCOL

Calculating Calories and Macronutrients (macros)

- Set grams of protein equal to lean body weight in pounds.
- Suggested starting macro percent is 30:40:30 (carbs, protein, fat).
- Calculate calories based on protein level (see examples).
- Walk 10–15K steps daily, and do no less than 3 intense workouts per week.
- Adjust calories and macros based on results and biofeedback.

Remember!
4 cal per gram of carbohydrate,
4 cal per gram of protein, 9 cal per gram of fat

185-Pound Female, 30% Fat

Set protein to 185 − (185 × 0.30) = 130g

130 × 4 cal = 520 cal protein

520 ÷ 0.40 = 1300 total cal

(1300 × 0.30 carbs) ÷ 4 cal = 98g carb

(1300 × .30 fat) ÷ 9 cal = 43g fat

1300 total cal
98g carb, 130g protein, 43g fat

240-Pound Male, 27% Fat

Set protein to 240 − (240 × 0.27) =175g

175 × 4 cal =700 cal protein

700 ÷ 0.40 = 1750 total cal

(1750 × 0.30 carbs) ÷ 4 cal = 131g carb

(1750 × 0.30 fat) ÷ 9 cal = 58g fat

1750 total cal
131g carb, 175g protein, 58g fat

The ELEL Intuitive Approach

Not everyone is a calorie counter or likes to obsess about macro-nutrient balance. For those types, it is fine to use a more intuitive or subjective starting place as it pertains to ELEL.

DIFFERENT WAYS TO ELEL

ELEL = eat less, exercise less. For those who exercise three or less times per week. For recovery from excess dietary stress, to minimize rebound weight gain and reduce metabolic compensation. Exercise is minimized, but slow walking and other stress reduction methods are emphasized.

Remember!

A very low-calorie diet without excess exercise
is not the same as one with excessive exercise.

CALORIES

Set Calories to 10 × body weight in pounds.

INTUITIVE	
3 : 2 : 1	**3** Meals per day
	2 Meals protein and vegetable only
	1 Meal includes starch and/or fat
	* Best in hours after workout

MACROS

· Set protein grams = lbs lean mass (LM)

· Macro ratio 30:40:30 (carbs, protein, fat)

· Back calculate total calories and macros

· Adjust up or down as needed based on results

Remember!

4 cal per gram carb

4 cal per gram protein

9 cal per gram fat

EXAMPLE

150-pound female, 20% body fat		1200 total cal
150 × 0.20 = 30 body fat	480 ÷ 0.40 = 1200 Total cal	90g carb
150 − 30= 120 protein grams (LM)	(1200 × 0.30) ÷ 4 = 90g carb	120g protein
120g × 4 = 480 cal protein	(1200 × 0.30) ÷ 9 = 40g fat	40g fat

Think of the macronutrient and calorie-specific calculations as an approach that begins by prioritizing the quantity of food. Think of the intuitive approach as leading with food quality.

The intuitive approach I like to use for ELEL is called the 3-2-1 approach. This is a system I devised over many years in the clinic to quickly and easily give people an introduction to quality nutrition. It's a formula that efficiently prescribes eating frequency along with quality targets for food. The first number, 3, designates how many meals or feeding opportunities the person will have daily. The second number designates the number of those meals that will be fat and starch reduced (i.e., consisting of only lean meats and vegetables). The last number is how many of the meals will include fat and/or starch. In this case, 3-2-1 means three meals daily, two without starch and fat, and one with fat and/or starch.

This same 3-2-1 designation can be used to quickly visualize what that last mixed meal should look like: three parts vegetable, two parts lean protein, and one part starch and/or fat.

As you can see, this is a very quick and easy approach to prescribe a metabolic meal plan that excels at calorie reduction, hunger control, and nutrient density. For those who hate counting, weighing, and measuring, it provides a solid beginning structure. If they are able to achieve results with it, there is no need to change this more intuitive approach to eating. However, if results are slow or nonexistent, moving to a more data-driven quantity tracking method may be necessary.

ELEL Exercise

Although ELEL is not a protocol that addresses exercise, it does not mean exercise can't be done. In fact, three weight training sessions or less per week help turn this protocol into a far more efficient fat loss toggle.

Doing three full-body weight training workouts per week on this protocol adds a mechanical stimulus and hormonal effect that help the body maintain lean muscle mass and accentuate fat loss. Exercise should not be emphasized in this toggle.

Walking is really the only thing required, but up to three weight training workouts per week are acceptable and may provide enhanced benefit.

Eat More, Exercise More

EMEM is the athlete toggle. Athletes need to eat enough to fuel their activities. No athlete in their right mind is going to eat less and exercise more if they want to perform and win at their sport. Athletes don't train to look good; they train to excel at the game they play. Looking good is just the natural outcome of a well-fueled body undergoing intense training. The idea that you can do ELEM to look like an athlete is absurd. Athletes don't starve themselves; rather, they eat more because they need to fuel their training. Eating less is not something that would aid athletic performance. In fact, it would impede it. It's why every few years when the Olympics roll around, you hear the commentators talking about the insane amount of food each athlete eats.

Whereas ELEL creates a calorie deficit with food, EMEM manipulates the calorie gap with exercise. The EMEM toggle is great for fat loss or muscle gain. If it is being used for fat loss, then exercise is ramped up to slightly exceed the amount that is being eaten. If it is being used to gain muscle, then exercise is kept just below the food intake so extra calories are driven toward muscle gain. Just as a calorie deficit and hormonal balance are required for fat loss, calorie excess and hormonal balance are required for muscle increases.

This toggle is not exclusive to professional athletes. Maybe you're someone who just loves to exercise. If that's the case, you have to up your calorie intake to compensate for the deficit. How much you up your intake will depend on the kind of exercise you do. For example, cardiovascular exercise burns the most calories while you're doing it. If you go for a run or take a spin class, you're going to burn a ton of calories, but the second you stop, so does the burning. There is no after effect. However, if you do weight training, you'll burn fewer calories during the actual session, but in the hours and days afterward, you are going to use energy to recover, repair muscle, and adapt by perhaps synthesizing new muscle.

This toggle also does not mean all you are allowed to eat is "health food." Food is fuel, and depending on your specific goals, you might need to introduce some "junk" food. For example, most people think a Snickers bar is an awful food, and I would agree that it is in *most* cases. But if you are starving, a Snickers bar is actually a health food. Similarly, people think broccoli is the best food on the planet. However, if you've already consumed 4,000 calories that day, broccoli is doing nothing for your health. If you eat an extra cup of broccoli at that point, all it does is add to your calorie load.

Furthermore, if you're an athlete who's burning massive amounts of energy, you can't only eat chicken and broccoli. You're simply not going to be able to get the number of calories you need. Even the hunter-gatherers of days past knew they needed things like fat and nuts for the energy they would provide. In today's world, things like peanut butter, cheeseburgers, pizza, and even candy bars can serve a purpose to an athlete. In fact, if you are going to include those things regularly in your diet, the EMEM toggle is the only appropriate way to do so. If you eat those things regularly while in any other toggle, they could end up stalling your progress.

EMEM is best done in blocks of eight to twelve weeks. When in EMEM, your calorie intake should be fifteen times your body weight in pounds.

Your macronutrient ratio should be 40 percent carbs, 30 percent protein, and 30 percent fat. Because carbs are like high-octane jet fuel for performance, the body will use the extra amount both to build muscle and fuel activities. If you're a hard gainer, meaning you are super lean and have a tough time gaining muscle, you may need to go as high as twenty times your body weight to determine your ideal calorie intake and set the macros to 40-30-30.

Keep in mind these ratios are just suggestions for a place to start. There is no magic in these formulas. You will still have to use the AIM process to analyze what your metabolism reacts to and make adjustments. Your body will tell you how many calories and macronutrients you need. You might end up with a 50-30-20 ratio. This structure exists only as a starting point; tweak it to reflect your unique needs.

EMEM Macronutrient Calculation

Like with ELEL, EMEM can be done in a very intuitive way or a very math-oriented way. Let's deal with the more specific quantity approach first. Remember, with EMEM, we want to elevate food intake in general and carbohydrate intake in particular. Intense athletic training requires a fueling strategy that includes more glucose. Although there has been a renewed interest in low-carbohydrate approaches to fueling sport over the last few years, almost all of the research in this direction has reaffirmed the primacy of glucose as a preferred performance fuel. The extra glucose is also a prime stimulant of insulin, which is arguably the most anabolic hormone in the body as cells don't get fed without it. These considerations are the reason EMEM adjusts the macronutrient ratio with higher carbohydrate levels of 40-30-30 carb, protein, and fat.

The simple and dirty way to calculate calories would be to use body weight times fifteen for the average person looking to fuel exercise while focusing on getting leaner (i.e., burning body fat). Scaling up to body weight times twenty would be for those most interested in gaining muscle.

Of course, as you have learned, these numbers are always just best starting places. The proof of the numbers will be apparent or not based on results. The EMEM approach can be used to create a calorie deficit for fat loss or a calorie surplus for muscle gain.

To get even more specific, protein again can be used as the basis for the calorie calculations. Given the strong demands on the metabolism for recovery and adaptation, protein levels should be elevated even further in the EMEM toggle. To account for this, I set the grams of protein to pounds of body weight. For example, I am 225 pounds. If I were to move into an EMEM toggle, 225 would be my target for grams of protein intake. From there, I can back-calculate to determine the calories and 40-30-30 macronutrient ratio:

- 225 pounds means my protein grams will be 225 grams.

- There are 4 calories per gram of protein, so I multiply 225 by 4, giving me 900 calories of protein.

- Next, I cross-multiply and divide 900 calories by .30, giving me a total calorie level of 3,000.

- From there, I can take 40 percent of 3,000 for the carbohydrate calories of 1,200. There are 4 calories per gram of carb, so 1,200 divided by 4 gives the grams of carbohydrate: 300 grams.

- I can do the same calculation for fat: 3,000 multiplied by 30 percent fat gives us 900 calories of fat. Fat has 9 calories per gram, so 900 divided by 9 is 100 grams of fat. This yields 3,000 calories at 300 grams carbs, 225 grams protein, and 100 grams fat.

If you are savvy, you will see one issue with doing calculations in this way. What if you are someone who is obese? Normally, an obese person will not be able to sustain the type of activity required for the EMEM protocol without putting themselves at risk for injury. But that is not a hard-and-fast rule. So to account for this, if I have someone greater than 30 percent body fat, I typically will not set protein grams any higher than 200 on the EMEM protocol.

This helps account for the excessive fat tissue and keeps the calorie levels down to a level more in line with what a leaner version of that person would be consuming. This saves us from excessive protein intake. We would not necessarily want someone 300 pounds consuming 300 grams of protein given that would require a calorie intake of 4,000 and possibly be excessive for fat loss goals. This underscores the need to always think about the uniqueness of each person. A lean 225-pound lifter is different than an obese

225-pound couch potato. This is why the ELEL protocol is usually preferred for the very obese. If EMEM is going to be used in these individuals, you are best to limit protein to 200 grams.

EAT MORE, EXERCISE MORE PROTOCOL
Calculating Calories and Macronutrients (macros)

- Set grams of protein equal to lean body weight in pounds.
- Suggested starting macro percent is 40:30:40 (carbs, protein, fat).
- Calculate calories based on protein level (see examples).
- Walk 10–20K steps daily, and do 4–7 intense workouts per week.
- Adjust calories and macros based on results and biofeedback.

Remember!
4 cal per gram of carbohydrate,
4 cal per gram of protein, 9 cal per gram of fat

140-Pound Athletic Female

Set protein to 140g

140 × 4 cal = 560 cal protein

560 ÷ 0.30 = 1866 total cal

(1866 × 0.40 carbs) ÷ 4 cal = 186g carb

(1866 × 0.30 fat) ÷ 9 cal = 62g fat

1866 total cal
186g carb, 140g protein, 62g fat

200-Pound Athletic Male

Set protein to 200g

200 × 4 cal = 800 cal protein

800 ÷ .30 = 2666 total cal

(2666 × 0.40 carbs) ÷ 4 cal = 267g carb

(2666 × 0.30 fat) ÷ 9 cal = 88g fat

2666 total cal
267g carb, 200g protein, 88g fat

The intuitive approach to EMEM follows the 4-2-2 formula: 4 meals per day, 2 with only lean protein and vegetables, and 2 mixed meals including starch and/or fat. The mixed meal plates would also follow half the plate being vegetables, a quarter being lean protein, and a quarter being starch or fat.

DIFFERENT WAYS TO EMEM

EMEM = eat more, exercise more. For those training intensely all or most days of the week. Also those looking to support athletic pursuits, gain muscle, or drive fat loss through activity.

CALORIES

Set Calories to 15 × body weight in pounds if desire weight loss.

INTUITIVE		
4 : 2 : 2	**4** Meals per day	
	2 Meals protein and vegetable only	
	2 Meal includes starch and/or fat	
	* Best in hours after workout	

MACROS

· Protein grams equal to lbs body weight

· Macro ratio 40:30:30 (carbs, protein, fat)

· Back calculate total calories and macros

· Adjust up or down as needed based on results

Remember!

4 cal per gram carb

4 cal per gram protein

9 cal per gram fat

EXAMPLE

200-pound male		2666 total cal
200g × 4 = 800 cal protein	(2666 × 0.40) ÷ 4 = 266g carb	266g carb
800 ÷ 0.30 = 2666 total cal	(2666 × 0.30) ÷ 9 = 89g fat	200g protein
		89g fat

EMEM Exercise

With EMEM, exercise is most definitely accentuated. For the EMEM toggle to be effective, at least four long duration and/or high-intensity workouts should be performed per week. Remember, this is an athletic protocol. Both movement and metabolics should be utilized. This is athletic training at its best, and the best exercise modalities will be those that utilize intense weight training and cardio. In the EMEM protocol, any type of exercise is game, but weight training should most definitely be the dominant form of metabolics in order to help the body maintain or even gain muscle while simultaneously burning fat.

Metabolism is not a great multitasker. It either likes to be burning muscle and fat or gaining muscle and fat. The EMEM protocol is the one that helps the metabolism multitask better. If you are looking to simultaneously gain muscle and burn fat, this is the protocol for you.

The Fifth Toggle: ESES

There is actually one more metabolic toggle that represents caloric equilibrium. You can think of this as a maintenance toggle. It's the metabolic state where the intake of calories and output of energy are relatively stable and balanced. This is referred to as isocaloric to distinguish it from hypocaloric (low-calorie state or deficit) and hypercaloric (high-calorie state or excess). Many people live in this ESES state and choose never to diet at all, living happily here. In fact, most of the people you see eating and exercising and being able to maintain that lifestyle year in and year out are actually in the ESES state NOT the ELEM state. This is a major point of confusion for people who look at others with healthy lifestyles and assume they are always eating less and exercising more. They are not. They are usually either in an EMEM athletic state and thereby creating a calorie deficit or excess for fat loss or muscle gain, respectively, or more likely they are in the ESES state.

You can think of ESES as your home base. It is the place that keeps your body weight stable and does not result in weight loss or weight gain. In fact, this is a very important toggle to understand as often losing substantial amounts of body fat requires a constant return to this balanced holding pattern of ESES. Remember that anytime there is a gap between calorie intake and output, it can possibly create more pressure on the metabolic stress barometer. Do that for too long and the metabolism will react negatively. However, spending only short periods of time in calorie deficits and then returning to isocaloric levels is one of the most effective strategies I have found clinically to get the weight off and keep it off.

This is also a major point of confusion and contention for coaches working with individuals for weight loss. These coaches will often rightly deduce that someone who is eating less and exercising more but not getting results needs to do something different. Often, their solution is to have them eat more and exercise less, moving them from one stressful metabolic toggle, ELEM, to another stressful metabolic toggle, EMEL.

Instead, they should be moving them into EMEM by simply having them eat more to match output or move them into ELEL by having them exercise less to match output. Or it could be even better to simply move them gently back to a diet and exercise approach where exercise, calories, and food intake are balanced out completely, or ESES. This is the best approach to take. This is my version of a "diet break" and avoids the consequences of the ELEM to EMEL switch.

This is the approach used in the often-quoted study on intermittent energy restriction called the MATADOR study (minimizing adaptive thermogenesis and deactivating obesity rebound).[26] The study compared two groups of people. Both groups were put through a calorie-reduced lifestyle of 30 percent. Each group followed the diet for sixteen weeks. The traditional diet group simply did continuous energy restriction for the entire time period. The other group dieted by taking two weeks in energy deficit followed by two weeks in an isocaloric state. In other words, one group did ELEM for sixteen weeks; the other did two weeks in ELEM followed by a two-week diet break in ESES for a total period of thirty-two weeks (sixteen of which were in ELEM, exactly the same as the control group). Both groups lost weight, but the intermittent group lost more weight, more fat, and less muscle. Weight loss was thirty-one pounds in the intermittent calorie restriction and twenty pounds in the continuous calorie restriction group. Fat loss was just shy of twenty-five pounds in the group taking diet breaks and seventeen pounds in the other group. After six months of not following any calorie restriction, the participants were checked again. The group alternating ELEM with ESES was still down eighteen pounds while the other group had regained all but five pounds.

Although this study was met with great fanfare when it first came out, studies done since have been mixed in terms of the effectiveness of this approach. That being said, long before the MATADOR study was published, this approach of diet breaks and alternating patterns of calorie intake versus output had already proven effective in my clinical work for at least a decade.

It is important when evaluating effective tools to be aware of both the art and the science of nutritional approaches. The art of nutritional science happens on the fringe of the research where existing understanding meets big gaps in our knowledge. It's in that chasm (i.e., the gap between what we know and what we don't know) where new ideas and tactics are explored. Often, these tools and techniques work in the clinic despite not yet having scientific support. This is why a savvy coach realizes that science only sometimes defines the approach; more often, it refines the approach.

TIMING IS EVERYTHING

As you'll have noticed by now, you should not stay in the ELEM or EMEL toggles for long periods of time. EMEM can be done for much longer but often requires breaks given it is a more grueling regime. ELEL and ESES are toggles that you can most certainly live in indefinitely. You actually should be jumping around between toggles, because as you do, your metabolism becomes more resilient and more flexible. As it becomes less and less rigid, you have freedom to bounce back and forth. For instance, when you stay in ELEL or EMEM for a few weeks, then jump to ELEM, you may actually see results again, albeit just for another short period of time. If you stay in one toggle for too long, your metabolism will inevitably adapt and results will cease. The more flexible you are about switching toggles, the more flexible your metabolism will be.

The easiest way to gauge when it's time to switch toggles is to listen to HEC and SHMEC. HEC and SHMEC are always the most efficient way to assess metabolic stress. However, you can also look for other cues as to when it's best to move from one to another. For example, women can choose toggles to coincide with their menstrual cycles. EMEM is an ideal choice when estrogen is dominating, whereas ELEL is best when progesterone is in charge (more on this in Chapter Eight).

You could toggle seasonally the way our hunter-gatherer ancestors did. In that scenario, winter is ideal for ELEL. Then, as the weather warms and animals emerging from a long winter are leaner, ELEM is the natural choice. That doesn't last long, however, because the foliage and food sources soon become more plentiful and you begin moving more, which means it's time for EMEM. The last weeks or so of late fall make the most sense for EMEL, as animals fatten up in anticipation of winter and days becoming shorter.

WHEN TO EMEM AND ELEL

EMEM: Eat More, Exercise More. Uses exercise to create calorie deficit. Can also be used when looking to gain muscle.

ELEL: Eat Less, Exercise Less. Uses food to create calorie deficit.

1 TRAINING-BASED

- EMEM on training days
- ELEL on recovery days
- Training days, eat more to fuel activity
- Non-training days, eat less and let the body fuel recovery, repair, and adaptation
- EMEM during heavy training blocks
- ELEL during recovery times

2 MENSES-BASED

- EMEM during follicular phase (first 2 weeks)
- ELEL during luteal phase (last 2 weeks)

  OR

- EMEM late follicular phase and early luteal phase (middle 2 weeks)
- ELEL late luteal phase and early follicular phase (week before and during menses)

3 TIME-BASED

- EMEM weekends
- ELEL weekdays
- 2 weeks in each
- 1 month on each
- EMEM summer and fall
- ELEL winter and spring
- Or any other variation

4 BIOFEEDBACK

- Switch protocols when HEC (hunger, energy, cravings) and other parameters go out of check
- Switch protocols when results stop
- Switch protocols when bored

You also can do it according to your workweek, when ELEL might make the most sense during the weekdays since you're not exercising and EMEM works better on the weekends when you are more active. Then, if you want to enjoy time with friends and family, you can do EMEL every once in a while.

Finally, the savviest fitness enthusiasts can use an ELEL style of eating on days where you are not working out and an EMEM style of eating on the days you do work out. In fact, many active individuals have naturally and intuitively adopted this approach, even using an intermittent fasting approach on the days they travel or are not very active.

Again, as is the case with all things metabolism, you have to do what's right for you when it's going to work best for you. Your body will send you the signs when it's time to switch things up, and by now, you should know how to look for them.

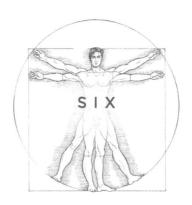

THE METABOLIC ATHLETE

E xercise is critical for metabolic health. From that perspective, it does not matter what you choose to do—
any type of exercise will have tremendous benefits for
your mood and your vitality. One thing that may be a
bit confusing, however, is the fact that healthy exercise is not the
same as fat loss exercise.

Obviously, covering all aspects of exercise would take several
books. Because this book is focused on optimizing metabolism
for fat loss, I am going to focus only on that aspect of exercise.

It's important to remember that what you like to do, what helps
your heart and mood, may not be helping you get the lean, athletic look you want. This chapter is meant to give you an updated

understanding of what it will take for you to get that very look most of us strive for. That look requires building and maintaining lean tissue (muscle) and losing fat. The lean athletic physique is not just the one most of us desire—it's also the healthiest thing for your metabolism. Optimizing body composition, the amount of muscle versus fat, is the best of all worlds. This helps you look good, feel good, live longer, and function better.

Before we get deeper into this, I need to clear up two pretty big misunderstandings most people have. The first is that most people believe if they exercise in a manner similar to their favorite athlete, they will achieve that same athletic look. The truth is that most athletes don't look the way they look because of the exercise they do; they do the exercise they do because of the way they look.

It is important to realize that most of those lean runners you see were lean before they started running. When they were introduced to the activity, they excelled, and it became their sport. That is not to say you won't ever meet a weightlifter who used to be skinny or a runner who used to be bulkier. It just means those types are far rarer. In the end, you need to do what research says works and what also adheres to your natural metabolic strengths. For some, that is going to mean far more weight training than cardio, and for others, a good mix of weight training and cardio.

The next big misunderstanding is to think that exercise is only about what it does during the activity. In reality, you need to be thinking about what exercise does not just during but also in the hours and days after exercise. If you are looking to optimize your muscle-to-fat ratio, then doing a 500-calorie workout that causes you to be so hungry you end up consuming 800 calories is not smart. In the same way that what you eat at one meal will influence what and how much you eat at the next meal, so too will the kind of exercise you do impact how much you eat and what you crave.

When it comes to exercise, you want to engage in the types of workouts that maximize calorie burn during activity, optimize hormonal balance after the workout, and do not have a negative impact on hunger and cravings. The science on what style of training does best in this regard is still being worked out, but we do have some hints about what may work best and what won't.

WEIGHT TRAINING

The single most important type of workout to do to attain and maintain optimal body composition is likely weight training for most. Lifting weights does not burn as many calories during the workout as an equivalent amount of cardio will. The benefits of weight training accrue after the workout is over. While you are weight lifting, you burn some calories. In the hours after a workout using weights, you will use more calories to recover from the workout. In the day after that, you will burn more calories as you repair the muscle damage the workout created.

In the day after that, even more energy is used to adapt by creating strong ligaments, tendons, and muscle.

When you do a cardiovascular activity, the afterburn of the workout is negligible. After resistance training, the postworkout calorie burn lasts for hours and days and can be substantial. In addition, weight lifting is the only type of activity that coaxes the body to use any extra calories for muscle growth rather than fat gain. It is the workout that keeps on giving.

The trick with weight training is to know how to do it right. Your metabolism has a way to measure the demand placed on it, and the greater that demand, the more it triggers downstream calorie use and adaptation processes. The triggers for muscle adaptation are the time a muscle remains under tension, the metabolic by-products that build up in and around that muscle, and the total volume of work that muscle is forced to do.

Volume, in this case, can be calculated by multiplying the weight by reps by sets that a muscle, or group of muscles, is subjected to. So if I am working out by doing a barbell back squat with a weight of 225 pounds and I do that for 5 sets of 10 reps, then the total volume the leg muscles have done is $225 \times 10 \times 5 = 11,250$. This "workload" is one of the things that muscle responds to and grows from. Of course, muscle adapts and so progressive overload is a huge component of effective weight lifting. Progressive overload is about increasing the amount of work (volume) muscles are exposed to. This means in a few weeks or months, the weight on the barbell back squats should be increased. Alternatively, the sets and reps can be adjusted. You can also make the workout "denser" by cramming the same volume into a shorter amount of time. All of these methods can increase the demand on the muscle in one of the three ways mentioned (metabolic demand, tension, and volume).

Effective weight training should be challenging enough to elicit a sizable recovery, repair, and adaptation response.

WORKOUT BIOFEEDBACK

There are four main biofeedback sensations to pay attention to during exercise. I call them the Bs and Hs (breathless, burning, heavy, and heat). Each of these biofeedback sensations has a host of metabolic and hormonal associations with it.

Breathlessness

Breathlessness is how the body responds to the increased demand for oxygen by the working muscles. In response to increased muscle activity, the body ramps up respiration and heart rate. It does this through the release of catecholamines (adrenaline and noradrenaline). These hormones have multiple mechanisms of action. They open up the airways in the lungs, they speed heart rate, and they help liberate glucose from the liver and fat from the adipose tissue. The point where these hormones kick in is right where talking in a workout becomes impossible. Lower intensity cardio workouts, where you can talk without difficulty, burn calories, but they miss some of these hormonal effects.

Ideally, an exercise will push your body hard enough that you will be breathless for a short time after. If you are conditioned for running and go for a jog, you could probably carry on a conversation with someone jogging next to you. If you were doing sprint intervals, on the other hand, running hard and fast for a certain distance, you and your workout partner would not be able to comfortably talk for a minute or two after. In fact, this kind of exertion is so intense that it demands you stop and take a breather for a time before you repeat the effort again.

Compared to steady-state cardio or old-fashioned aerobics, such as that done in a step class, spin workout, or jogging, sprint intervals elicit much greater demand on the system per unit time, are more likely to create the hormonal adrenaline release, and will boost post-exercise calorie burn significantly.

What many don't realize is that a heavy set of weight lifting can produce the exact response sprinting does, especially when the exercise is a full-body movement like squats. One of the reasons individuals who lift heavy weights must drop the weights, stop, and rest is because it would be impossible to keep going under such intensity. Weight training can be a lot like intervals or sprint training, especially with the right intensity.

Burning

Burning in the muscle is another indication of intensity. As muscle works, mitochondria (the cell's energy factory) are busy chopping up carbon compounds from the food you have eaten or stored and generating protons (hydrogen atoms). These protons create an energy gradient across the mitochondrial membranes, and this charge is used to make the body's energy packet, ATP.

In ultrademanding conditions, mitochondrial shuttles (that bring protons to the inner mitochondria, compounds like NADH and FADH2) become "maxed out" like a subway car at full capacity. Once that occurs, protons start building up in the cell, causing the pH of the cell to become more acidic. These changes cause the muscle to be less efficient and begin to fatigue and also cause a burning sensation in the muscle. To buffer against the pH change, the cell uses lactate to grab hold of protons. Lactate then becomes lactic acid.

Many people believe lactic acid is causing the burning in the muscle, but in reality, it is buffering against it. Lactic acid is a nifty compound for the body because the cell can use it to make energy and export it to other surrounding cells for their energy use as well.

It has also been demonstrated in mice that lactic acid acts as a signaling molecule that may be a major trigger of human growth hormone. So whereas breathlessness is an indication of sympathetic drive and adrenaline release, burning is an indication of HGH release. HGH is a hormone that aids recovery through ramping up fat use, suppressing muscle breakdown, aiding collagen repair, and working with testosterone to build lean tissue.

Just like with breathlessness, burning and the fatigue that accompanies it can't be sustained for long and therefore requires the exerciser to rest briefly to recover so they can achieve the same intensity once again. Burning is an indicator the muscle is under high metabolic stress. One of the other things that occurs in muscle subjected to this kind of intense work is the release of myokines.

Myokines are signaling molecules. Many of these muscle molecules are also used by the immune system to regulate inflammation and infection responses. When these compounds are released from immune cells, we call them cytokines. When they are released from the muscle, they are called myokines. If you want an easier way to think of them, just think of them as metabolic smoke. When the muscles are burning, they release this myokine "smoke."

Myokines produced by a muscle are released and send signals to other muscles close by. But they also send signals to the brain that influence appetite. They go to the fat cells and influence fat release. They go to the liver and influence fuel partitioning, and they go to the gut and immune cells for cross-talk there.

I don't want to make this a biochemistry lesson, but it is useful to know that this kind of intense muscular work has many benefits, including this myokine response. Some of the more important of these compounds are IL-6, IL-15, and IL-8.

IL-6 is often thought of as an inflammatory compound, but when it is released from the muscles, it has a different impact, suppressing inflammatory compounds like TNF and IL-1 and triggering anti-inflammatory compounds like IL-10. It also may suppress appetite and ramp up fat burning. IL-15 is a muscle-building molecule. IL-8 triggers the growth of new blood vessels.

Again, exercise is not simply about burning calories—it also signals a sophisticated array of messages that help you get leaner, faster, stronger, and more muscular. This is the reason athletes look and function the way they do.

Certain types of exercise excel at these effects, and certain types are simply about calorie burning. To develop a lean athletic physique, you want both the calorie-burning and hormonal effects of exercise on your side.

Heavy

Heavy is all about creating strain and tension through the muscles and joints. The heavy component is about the load the working muscles are subjected to. This is a very straightforward biofeedback sensation and it is associated with the testosterone effect of weight training. Testosterone is a hormone that aids lean muscle gain and ramps up fat burning. Not to sound like a broken record, but in order to lift the loads required to get significant testosterone effects, rest between sets is crucial.

Many individuals pick up weights they can lift 50 or 100 times. To get the testosterone effect, you really want to hit the sweet spot, which research hints might sit right around the 8–12 rep zone or what we call a 10-rep max (10RM). A 10-rep max is a weight you can complete 10 times but not 11. In order to work with these weights, it requires adequate recovery of one to three minutes of rest. If the rest is too short, muscle recovery is inadequate and achieving all the reps is less likely.

HORMONAL BIOFEEDBACK IN EXERCISE

The type of exercise you do determines the hormonal outcome of the workout and the metabolic outcome and body change results.

Pay attention to the biofeedback sensations of breathlessness, burning, heavy, and heat.

Breathless	**Adrenaline, Cortisol**
Burning	**HGH, Testosterone**
Heavy	**Testosterone, HGH**
Heat	**Sympathetic Activation**

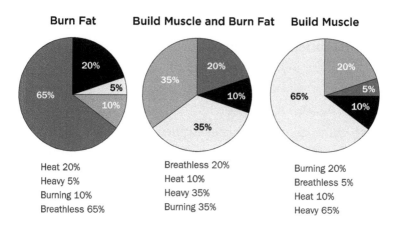

Burn Fat

Heat 20%
Heavy 5%
Burning 10%
Breathless 65%

Build Muscle and Burn Fat

Breathless 20%
Heat 10%
Heavy 35%
Burning 35%

Build Muscle

Burning 20%
Breathless 5%
Heat 10%
Heavy 65%

Heat

Thermal challenge is another adaptation response. When the body's core temperature rises, it will induce a sweating response to try to cool off. The more you sweat, the more thermal challenge the body is encountering. This sweat response, like the breathless response, is triggered by the sympathetic nervous system (fight/flight response). So when sweating kicks in, it is a good indication that the adrenaline response is adequate.

Thermal challenges also do more. The release of chaperone proteins, called heat shock proteins, is a hallmark of heat exposure. Chaperone proteins do exactly what they sound like—they hang out around other proteins and help them out. Chaperone proteins help other body proteins maintain their three-dimensional structure. That structure is directly related to how well a protein does its job.

Heat surges in the body also activate what are known as transcription factors. A transcription factor helps turn certain genes on and others off. In the case of thermal challenge from exercise, the genes turned on are the ones that increase brain growth factors, regulate inflammation, optimize body composition, and more.

REST IS SUCCESS

Rest and work are not opposites; they are synergists. All those biofeedback sensations mentioned above require rest in order to be achieved again and again. Remember the theme of fat loss? Burning off fat and keeping it off requires two things: calorie deficits and an optimal hormonal state of function.

When we talked about the 4Ms of metabolism (mindfulness, movement, meals, and metabolics), I mentioned that exercise (metabolics) was probably the least important of the four for beginners and even most people trying to lose weight. The reason is that exercise speeds up metabolism and can trigger hunger and cravings.

The shorter the workout, the less likely that is to happen. However, if we are going to achieve results from exercise, a shorter workout necessitates a more intense workout. And when intensity goes up, rest must be used.

One of the things I am known for in the fitness world is the development of rest-based training (RBT). The concept is based on a simple question: because we need more-intense workouts and because every person has a different level of fitness and physical abilities, how can we personalize the workout to give the exact intensity needed based on the individual? The answer is to give everyone the same style of workouts, but let them rest whenever and for however long they need in the workout.

The mantra to remember is "push until you can't and rest until you can." As you have learned, intense exertion is the major determinant of physical adaptation while rest is the chief driver of intensity. Without rest, exercise must be naturally regulated with pacing strategies. This is a key insight because aerobic exercise modalities by their very nature do not employ rest. With aerobic exercise, the only options to increase intensity are going farther or exercising longer. This may not be the most efficient way to drive results.

CARDIO IS NOT CUTTING IT

And one of the most depressing studies on aerobic exercise shows that a full 75 percent of individuals using cardio training to attempt weight loss (with as much as forty-five minutes five days a week) see no weight loss at all.

In fact, only 25 percent of individuals seem to get any weight loss with these modalities and another 25 percent actually end up getting fatter as a result of cardio driving them to overcompensate with food.

At the same time, researchers have determined that higher intensity exercise like weight training and interval exercise burns significantly more calories than once thought and can provide a substantial metabolic advantage.[27] Anaerobic contributions to energy use can be underestimated by 70 percent for weight training and 95 percent for interval exercise.[28] The metabolic advantage can also result in a significant "afterburn" that can last sixteen hours in women and forty-eight hours in men.[29]

Interval training, boot camps, metabolic conditioning, and other more anaerobic programs may be better choices than straight cardio programs. These approaches are more likely to achieve the Bs and Hs discussed. They also seem to deliver on the promise of results. When compared head-to-head against traditional aerobics, some research shows substantial benefit. One study looked at a twenty-minute anaerobic interval program compared to forty minutes of aerobics. The programs were conducted three times each week for fifteen weeks. At the end of the study, the anaerobic group lost approximately five pounds of fat while the aerobic group showed a nonsignificant trend toward fat gain.[30]

The trick is to adopt some of the tools and techniques of higher intensity exercise protocols while keeping the workouts safe and scalable for all fitness levels. This is not an easy task. The average exerciser is not always equipped physiologically or psychologically to push themselves to the exertion levels required to generate the results they seek. Rest-based training solves this issue.

EXERCISE, MOTIVATION,
AND SELF-REGULATION

Rest-based training draws inspiration from the school of psychology and its self-determination theory (SDT).[31] Self-determination theory posits that those who are given autonomy over change are far more likely to develop and maintain innate motivation. This is in contrast to those who are coerced into change. Rest-based training brings this concept to exercise. By giving the exerciser control over when to rest and for how long, work volume can increase while safety is maintained.

Many current exercise trends work against the principles of self-determination theory. The keep-up militancy of boot camps and the competitive approach of some metabolic conditioning programs are prime examples. These approaches, although effective for some, may be counterproductive for significant segments of the population.

RBT flips these models around and gives complete control of the workout over to the exerciser. By doing so, it creates self-motivation and ownership over exercise so that participants not only work harder but also become better aware of their physiology and more engaged in their programs. RBT encourages participants to adjust work and rest ratios according to their individual needs. This is where the "push until you can't, rest until you can" concept comes in.

Contrary to popular perception, exercisers given the ability to self-regulate exertion do not necessarily default to lower exercise intensities. A review by Panteleimon Ekkekakis, a professor of exercise psychology at Iowa State University, highlights research showing that exercisers instead work at greater intensities than predicted.[32] This remains true so long as the intensity remains below the anaerobic threshold. This is the whole theory behind interval training, which employs rest to allow greater exertion. RBT takes this concept one step further by using rest coupled with control. This achieves the results of interval training while keeping the workout safe and appropriate for all fitness levels.

Self-regulation in exercise is a built-in feature of movement management seen in animals. Animals naturally regulate exercise by using a burst-then-rest strategy. This is likely an evolutionary adaptation allowing animals to maximize distances covered in a given time. It appears humans have the same ability to regulate intensity by employing rest.

REST-BASED TRAINING VERSUS INTERVAL TRAINING

The main goal of interval training is to balance the work intensity of every interval using the help of rest. Implementing the shortest rest period possible for metabolic recovery helps accomplish this. The "metabolic recovery" has to do with the clearance of hydrogen ions, restoration of phosphocreatine, recycling of lactate, and resetting of electrolyte gradients. Once this is accomplished, the physiology can perform at a high level once more. This reset point is likely different for everyone.

Definitive interval protocols can present challenges. Intervals like thirty seconds of work followed by thirty seconds of rest are often too intense for the average exerciser and provide inadequate metabolic recovery. At best, this will cause pacing that compromises workout results, and at worst, presents safety concerns.

According to RBT, individuals will self-regulate work and rest intervals to maximize intensity and ensure adequate recovery. Research shows this is indeed the case. In a 2010 study, eleven well-trained runners were put through two trials. In the first trial, one, two, and four minutes of rest were given after four minutes of intense exertion. Researchers wanted to determine which resting protocol provided adequate metabolic reset for the physiology. They found one minute was too short, four minutes was too long, and two minutes was just right.

The experiment was then repeated. Only this time, the exercisers were instructed to rest as long as they felt was adequate and then resume the workout when they "felt" ready.

Surprisingly, the average rest taken by the participants in the second experiment was 118 seconds, almost identical to the two minutes researchers previously determined was most beneficial from a physiological perspective.

The researchers concluded, "The concept of self-pacing facilitates greater self-awareness of physical capabilities…and it is our contention that the combination of using ratings of perceived exertion to gauge interval effort and perceived readiness scales to gauge recovery may be a useful means of organizing interval training according to individual conditioning requirements."[33]

REST-BASED TRAINING PRINCIPLES

The four key components of RBT are represented by the acronym REST:

- **R = Rest based**. Rest, not work, is the goal of rest-based training. This automatically increases the quality of work done, and it makes exercise psychologically easier. When exercisers have permission to rest according to their needs, they voluntarily work harder without being consciously aware they are doing so.[34]

- **E = Extrinsic focus**. Intrinsic sensations, such as breathlessness, burning, and other sensations, are inhibitors of exercise intensity. Rest-based training incorporates techniques that focus exercisers on what they are doing (extrinsic factors) versus what they are feeling (intrinsic feelings). With this in mind, an RBT workout is often structured to be quick moving and psychologically motivating.[35]

- **S = Self-determined**. RBT workouts are structured, but the exerciser has complete autonomy over exertion and rest. They are taught to use their rest strategically to push harder than they could without it.

  Giving control to the exerciser increases workout quality, improves exercise adherence, makes exercise psychologically easier, and improves results over time when compared to more definitive exercise prescriptions.

- **T = Time conscious**. Time and intensity are linked. So harder workouts must be shorter by necessity. RBT workouts usually last from twenty to forty minutes and incorporate start and stop working and resting segments according to individual needs.

RBT *in Practice*

To help the novice exerciser tap into their inherent ability to self-regulate exercise, RBT teaches a one-to-four scale. This scale works as both an exertion score and a readiness rating. It works to help the exerciser and/or their trainer recognize more clearly when they should rest and when they may want to resume training. Research has shown this to be a reliable tool in maximizing work and rest to generate optimal intensities for results.[36] It also keeps the workout safe and manageable.

RBT EXERTION SCALE

1. Exerciser is at rest.
2. Exerciser is exercising but can still talk, there is no burning in muscles, and/or the weight is light.
3. Exerciser can no longer talk, there is burning in the muscle, and/or the weight is getting heavy.
4. Exerciser must rest and recover.

RBT READINESS SCALE

1. Ready for full exertion.
2. Ready to attempt full exertion.
3. Unable to attempt full exertion.
4. No exertion is possible.

The goal of the workout is to reach a four on the RBT exertion scale repeatedly. Rest is then taken until the exerciser reaches a two on the RBT readiness scale. In time, the scales are no longer required as the participant learns to quickly home in on their self-regulating abilities.

RESISTANCE TRAINING

Resistance training using barbells, dumbbells, body weight, or other tools (kettlebells, bands, etc.) is the original rest-based workout. Most individuals do weight training in a very intuitive fashion, pushing themselves during their sets and then resting for as long as is required for them to exert maximum effort once more. For most people, this takes between one and five minutes of rest.

There are a few considerations here. Obviously, if your goal is to get as strong as possible, such as for a powerlifting competition, the loads lifted will be maximal and the rest taken will be prolonged. In this case, the heavy aspect of the Bs and Hs is being accentuated at the expense of breathlessness, burning, and heat.

If you shrink the rest periods down a little bit and lighten the loads to moderately heavy, such as the bodybuilding approach, then you are accentuating both heavy and burning, with much less breathlessness (except during the exertion) and heat.

If you shrink the rest periods down even more, you are able to equally institute all the Bs and Hs as the breathless component kicks into gear. This last approach can be thought of as "lifting weights faster." Not faster in the sense of lifting speed, but faster in the breathless sense of less rest between sets. This is more in line with metabolic conditioning that dominates the worlds of group exercise and CrossFit.

All of these methods are valid and each can have beneficial impacts on the metabolic adaptations we discussed in regard to weight lifting so long as they generate adequate intensity and continue to challenge the body through increased overload week after week. A study published in February 2021 in the *Journal of Sports Medicine and Physical Fitness* compared traditional weight training, CrossFit, and a popular group exercise lifting program called Les Mills Body Pump. The participants used these workouts five days a week for sixteen weeks. All showed benefit with traditional weight training and CrossFit showing enhanced effects on strength.[37] The point here is that weight training is essential and there are many ways to get the job done.

Part of the reason many people don't get the benefits they want from strength training is that they have never learned to understand how effective weight lifting feels. This is where the Bs and Hs come in and are so critical. Effective weight training will push the body in all four parameters but most importantly with burning and heavy. Don't turn your weight training into a cardio endeavor. Choose weight, set, rep, and rest schemes that get the muscle straining and burning.

CARDIO, YOGA, AND OTHER MODALITIES

There is nothing wrong with cardio—it is certainly exceedingly healthy. It has also been shown to be the best of all exercise modalities in terms of mood enhancement. There are those who will get amazing results with purely cardio-based exercise. The thing to remember, however, is that most people who do cardio by itself and have the athletic physiques to go along with it probably are suited to those activities and likely never had weight gain frustrations in the first place. This is not true of all cardio junkies, but in my thirty years in this field, I can count on one hand the number of overweight individuals who picked up a cardio-dominated exercise habit and became lean and athletic as a result. It simply rarely happens.

The same goes for yoga.

Yoga can in some people be incredibly intense and elicit some of the responses we talked about here, but like discussed previously, most yoga practitioners who have lean athletic bodies and excellent flexibility had those tendencies to begin with. As with purely cardio-dominated exercise, I have seen very few people take up yoga, Pilates, and other types of activity and get the bodies they wanted.

This underscores the need to always include what you love to do, but also make sure you know what is effective as well.

When it comes to cardio, we do need to get some myths out of the way. Cardiovascular exercise does indeed raise cortisol levels—so does every single other type of intense exercise. The only type of movement that lowers cortisol is relaxing movement. Slow walking, tai chi, yin-type yoga, MELT, and so forth. All of these can lower cortisol. Everything else raises it.

This is because cortisol is a stress hormone and is an acute response element of the body. It helps release blood sugar and fat to fuel working muscle in the same way adrenaline does. You don't want cortisol low during exercise; you want it high.

Cardiovascular exercises like running, biking, and the rest elevate cortisol the same way weight lifting does. The difference is that it does not also have the same impact on growth hormone and testosterone that weight lifting has. Hormones are like people; they behave differently depending on whom they are socializing with. When cortisol is elevated by itself or socializing with insulin, it can be a destructive muscle-wasting and fat-storing hormone. Cortisol amplifies the body's number one fat-releasing enzyme called HSL but also increases the body's number one fat-storing enzyme called LPL. In other words, cortisol is both a fat-storing and fat-releasing hormone.

When it is socializing with insulin, its HSL activity is blunted and its LPL activity is added to.

Fat storing is more likely if calorie intake is also high. On the other side, testosterone and growth hormones work against cortisol's LPL effects and accentuate its HSL effects, turning it into more of a fat burner if calories are also reduced.

The reason I bring this up is so you can understand if cardio is working for you or not. Cortisol also has the effect of stimulating the reward centers in the brain while decreasing the motivation centers. There is plenty of indication that it may also be implicated in the drive for highly palatable, calorie-rich food. In other words, cortisol goes hand in hand with cravings.

EXERCISE, HUNGER, AND CRAVINGS

There is abundant research showing that a very high percentage of individuals are not able to lose weight with exercise due to how that exercise triggers compensatory hunger and cravings.

These exercise-eating reactions are highly individualized. Not everyone will get these effects. That's also part of the reason why research in this area shows mixed results. Anytime you see an area of metabolic research that gives inconclusive outcomes, the law of metabolic individuality is likely at play. I have already taught you how to use HEC and SHMEC to determine if exercise is having a negative impact on you or not. However, intensity and duration have a lot to do with how your body responds to exercise. The longer and more intense the workout, the more compensatory eating reactions will likely be an issue. This is why I often try to keep my workouts more intense and also try to make them shorter.

Long, intense workouts and long, moderate workouts in the 60- to 120-minute range may be the worst offenders and trigger hunger and cravings more reliably.

Short, intense workouts in the 10- to 40-minute range usually have an acute appetite-suppressing effect (they can even make you feel nauseous) followed by hunger and craving amplification later. This short-term reduction in the drive to eat provides a preemptive strategy to get healthier foods on board before you start to crave the unhealthy stuff. This is why so many successful fitness enthusiasts often include a protein shake or meal replacement within an hour after intense workouts. It's about controlling hunger later.

When it comes to managing hunger and exercise, remember that the longer you are going to go, the slower you need to go. Slow walking, even done for a couple of hours, does not have the same hunger and craving triggering response. Turn that into a power walk or a jog and the outcome will be different.

Your best bet to get the results you want without compensatory eating is always to walk as much as is feasible, but exercise only just enough and do so using shorter, more intense modalities most of the time.

CARDIO AND MUSCLE

Another common concern is that cardiovascular exercise strips muscle off the body. This is not a reality for most people. In fact, what research shows is that strict calorie-reduced diets can result in near 20 percent of weight lost being in the form of lean body mass (water, muscle, organ tissue, etc.). Any type of activity that utilizes muscle, including running, acts as a resistor against this process. In other words, dieting without any exercise at all is what is going to cause muscle loss. Adding running will reduce that muscle loss. Adding weight training can result in no muscle loss at all and even muscle gain. And as far as the metabolism is concerned, that is the best of all worlds in terms of looking good, feeling good, living longer, and functioning better.

Another thing many people are surprised to hear is how well weight training and cardiovascular exercise aid each other. Cardio helps burn more fat when paired with weight training and weight training keeps cardio from burning off muscle. In other words, they are perfectly synergistic.

In the old days, this meant using several techniques. Doing weight lifting one day and cardio the next. Or using what is known as concurrent training where cardio was done first in the workout followed by weight training or vice versa. Both of those methods can be time intensive. This is where metabolic conditioning comes in. In this style of training, cardio and weight training are merged into one workout.

These metabolic conditioning workouts come in many flavors. When you are evaluating them, remember the rules of weight lifting—you want the heavy and burning effect in your muscles.

Don't turn these workouts into an exercise in breathlessness. The best way to do that is to simply shorten the rest periods of your lifting bouts in a "lift weights faster" mentality. This will generate the breathless response without needing any cardio type of exercises at all. This approach is the perfect way to merge cardio and weights in a very time-efficient manner.

TRADITIONAL WEIGHT LIFTING PROGRAM

Weight training is the number one modality for a lean athletic physique. Still, many people don't realize what effective weight lifting is. I also know not everyone likes this stuff. I get it. At the same time, there are just certain things that work better than others. So, by all means, do the exercise you love. Just realize that the thing we love is not always the thing that will get us results. If it's any consolation, I hate exercise in general. I have never done a workout I like. I do it because of how it makes me feel afterward, and I do it because it works.

A big hint is to stop treating breathlessness as the measure of a good workout.

If you want to magnify the hormonal and calorie-burning response in the hours and days after a workout, think about overloading your muscle. Here are two techniques that can make all the difference. Remember the way these techniques feel and try to reproduce them in your workouts.

The 10-Rep Max (10RM). Most people don't know what a heavy weight feels like. The 10RM will teach you. Choose any full-body exercise. I like the barbell back squat to illustrate.

Do a few warm-up sets. Go light. Then moderately heavy. Then aim for a weight you think you could do 10 of but not 11 (that's a 10RM). This will be hard and take all the mental and physical effort you can muster. In reality, you likely won't get it exactly at first. But go just shy of completing another rep. If you can't get 8, you went too heavy. Got more than 12? That's too light.

Now take a two- to three-minute rest. I know many people love being breathless, and you will be—only it will feel more like a sprint. When you train this heavy and intense, it becomes impossible to do anything else but focus on the task at hand, and like I said, that rest is crucial. Now do that for five more sets! That gives you an idea of how traditional weight training feels; don't make it any more complicated than that.

If you are a beginner to weight lifting, one to three full-body workouts a week is where you should start. This is known as a three-day full-body split. Use compound exercises that use multiple muscles and joints.

I recommend barbell back squat, barbell bench press, barbell deadlift, and barbell shoulder press. If you don't have barbells, dumbbells are fine. If you prefer machines, that's fine, too. What's more important is sticking to 3–5 sets of 8–12 reps of each exercise. Do exactly the same workout one to three times per week for eight to twelve weeks. This may seem boring, but remember, the metabolism does not care about such considerations.

There are things that work best and this is it. Besides, the adventure and interest come from seeing the improvement in weights lifted week after week.

Progressive overload is critical in all weight lifting. Progressive overload is often illustrated by the story of Milo of Croton. Milo was the strongest man in Greece, so the story goes.

BEGINNERS WEIGHT-TRAINING PROGRAMMING

- Train 3x per week
- Same workout all 3 days
- Take at least one day off between lifting sessions
- 4 full-body exercises
- 3–5 sets of each move
- 8–12 reps each set
- Can't do 8? Go lighter
- Can do more than 12? Go heavier
- 2–3 min between exercises
- Raise weight progressively
- Repeat 8–12 weeks
- Do NOT alter workout

- Variety is a results killer for beginners
- Stick to the basic moves
- Don't eat like an asshole

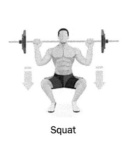

Squat

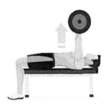

Bench press

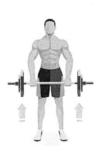

Deadlift

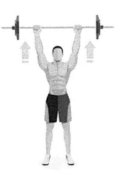

Shoulder press

He was given a baby calf when he was a young man, and every day he would hoist the calf to his shoulders and walk around with it. As the calf grew, Milo's muscles got stronger and stronger. One day, that baby calf was a full-grown cow weighing over 1,200 pounds and Milo could still pick it up. Although we can speculate on the limits of human strength and parables such as this, it does illustrate a point that everyone looking to develop a fit, lean body needs to remember: the body only responds with increasing demands.

Once they have three to nine months of training under their belts, many people graduate to a four-day split when upper and lower body exercises are separated: Monday and Thursday are upper and Tuesday and Friday are lower. Wednesday, Saturday, and Sunday are days off. Of course, any combination of three days off and four days on is fine. You get the point. This intermediate approach usually uses mostly compound exercises with a few accessories thrown in, like this:

- Upper: Barbell bench press 5 sets of 8–12. Barbell bent-over row 5 sets of 8–12. Dumbbell shoulder press 5 sets of 8–12. Tricep presses 3 sets of 8–12. Barbell bicep curl 3 sets of 8–12.

- Lower: Barbell back squat 5 sets of 8–12. Stiff-leg deadlift 5 sets of 8–12. Dumbbell walking lunges 5 sets of 8–12. Dumbbell step-ups 5 sets of 8–12. Calf raises 5 sets of 8–12.

Finally, the very advanced lifters often split the body up further and start to do more isolated exercises. This is the realm of bodybuilder splits and includes the five- and six-day splits. The five-day split is Monday through Friday lifting with the weekend off.

INTERMEDIATE WEIGHT-TRAINING WORKOUT

- Train 4 times per week
- Upper Body: Mondays and Thursdays
- Lower Body: Tuesdays and Fridays
- Wednesday, Saturday, Sunday off
- 4–5 full-body exercises per workout
- 1–2 isolation exercises per workout

- 3–5 sets of 8–12 reps each exercise
- Can't do 8? Go lighter
- Can do more than 12? Go heavier
- Raise weight progressively each week
- 2–3 min rest between exercises
- Repeat same workouts 8–12 weeks

Upper Body

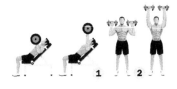

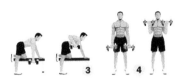

Lower Body

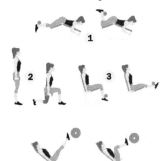

The six-day split takes only one day off. Because the body parts are staggered, the volume of each muscle is enhanced while recovery is attended to. These splits resemble something like the following:

- Monday—Chest and back
- Tuesday—Legs and core
- Wednesday—Shoulders and arms
- Thursday—Chest and back
- Friday—Legs and core
- Saturday—Off (five-day split) or shoulders and arms (six-day split)
- Sunday—Off

The point of all of this is that as one matures as a "lifter," the volume of the muscular work done per week may need to increase. Moving from a three- to four- and then five- or six-day split is one way to amplify the volume.

REST-BASED METABOLIC CONDITIONING

The reasons people don't engage in exercise are pretty clear. The number one cited reason is lack of time. After that, it's lack of know-how. This is where efficient exercise comes in. Metabolic conditioning workouts are perhaps the best of all worlds when it comes to getting the most bang for your buck with limited time.

Using the rest-based training approach I described earlier allows you to engage in very intense workouts that fit your individual fitness level exactly. The idea is to use weight lifting as the dominant activity, shorten the rest, and achieve the Bs and Hs all in one workout.

These workouts feel like interval training with weights and the results can be pronounced.

Here is a simple rest-based training workout called the Spark workout. It is by far the most popular and easy-to-implement workout I have ever written about. It was highlighted in my first book, *The Metabolic Effect Diet*, over ten years ago. It is still the most efficient workout I can teach you. Versions of this workout are now done by over a million individuals who have bought my online workout programs (Metabolic Aftershock, Metabolic Prime, and Metabolic Renewal).

You first need to understand what a compound exercise and a hybrid exercise are. A compound exercise is a weight lifting movement that uses multiple muscles and joints. A squat is a compound exercise because it uses the entire lower body (legs, butt, low back) and involves the ankle, knee, hip, and spine. A hybrid exercise combines two exercises into one. A squat followed by a curl and then a shoulder press is an example.

Here is how to construct a Spark workout:

- Choose four compound or hybrid exercises.

- There are two ways to set your weights. Choose a twenty-rep max on each exercise *or* choose a twelve-rep max for the exercise that is easiest of the four and use that same weight for all other moves.

- Set a timer for twenty minutes (roughly five minutes per exercise; if you chose five or six exercises, it would be twenty-five and thirty minutes, respectively).

- Complete twelve reps of each exercise in circuit fashion.

- Work until rest is required, then rest as long as needed before starting right where you left off.

- Continue this way, starting and stopping according to your own needs. Again, the mantra to remember is, "Push until you can't, rest until you can."

- Remember, there is no structured rest. The clock continues to run whether you are working or resting.

- When the clock time expires, the workout is done. Record how many rounds and reps you completed. Try to beat that time next time.

RULES:

- Choose 4 full-body exercises (use dumbbells, barbells, machines, or body weight)
- Do 12 reps and go to next exercise
- Do each exercise one after the other in circuit fashion
- Rest when you need to, then start again right where you left off (i.e., rest-based style)
- As many rounds/reps as possible for 20 minutes

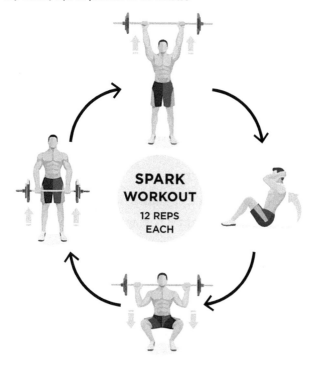

People will approach these workouts differently. Some will use lots of short rests while others will prefer less frequent and longer rests. Still others may use a combination of longer rests and shorter rest. Remember, just like with diet, do what works for you. In these workouts, you are only ever competing with yourself.

Here is an example metabolic conditioning workout fitting the above criteria:

- Dumbbell squat and press, dumbbell lunge and curl, push-ups, bent-over row.

- Push-ups and bent-over rows are great compound exercises targeting the chest and back. Those are paired with two hybrid exercises that tax the legs, shoulders, and arms.

- This is a workout that can be done three times per week for eight to twelve weeks. Yes, the same workout. Raise the weights each time and/or try to complete more reps in the time given.

You could also build other similar workouts if you get bored doing the same workout again and again. Just keep in mind that too much variation is counterproductive. Remember, we want progressive overload. You can't be progressive if you are changing the workout every single time.

EMEM AND ELEL

Eat more, exercise more (EMEM) and eat less, exercise less (ELEL) are admittedly vague terms. How much exercise should you do in these different metabolic toggles? Here is a general guide:

For ELEL, whether you are using traditional weight lifting or metabolic conditioning, one to three workouts a week is the limit. Extra cardio is discouraged. Only walking combined with lifting qualifies as ELEL.

For EMEM, four to seven workouts a week. In this case, all exercise modalities are game. I suggest four or five weight lifting or metabolic conditioning workouts per week along with two or three cardio sessions per week.

ELEM (eat less, exercise more) combines the eating strategy of ELEL with the workout approach of EMEM. Most dieters know this approach well. Keep in mind it should be done for only brief periods of one or two weeks max.

BUILDING COMPLEX WORKOUTS

One final consideration here is for those exercise enthusiasts who are building complex, multiple-element fitness programs. Where do mobility and stretching fit in with skill development along with cardio and weights?

I like to break these workout attributes down into strength, stamina, skill, and suppleness. Strength is the use of weights, stamina is the cardio component, skill is for mastering certain techniques (e.g., gymnastics, powerlifting exercises, etc.), and suppleness is about adding to body mobility and stability.

The easiest way to do this is to engage in metabolic conditioning workouts that deliver the Bs and Hs at the same time. This gives you the strength and stamina piece. You can then add on ten minutes for each of the skill and suppleness elements. These endeavors are great to use as warm-ups to your workout.

You also could break these up into different days like this:

- Monday—Suppleness and strength upper
- Tuesday—Suppleness and cardio
- Wednesday—Suppleness and upper body skill
- Thursday—Suppleness and lower body strength
- Friday—Powerlifting (skill)
- Saturday—Suppleness
- Sunday—Suppleness

You of course could combine these any way you want. Suppleness can also be achieved with other fitness modalities such as yoga, mobility workouts, foam rolling, and so on.

I encourage you to take on any of these workout recommendations and pay close attention to how they move you toward your desired outcomes. Remember, it's not about forcing yourself to do something simply because it's worked for others. The most important thing is to find what works best for you, your goals, and your metabolic health.

HOW TO MANAGE MIXED CONDITIONING PROGRAMS

Mixed conditioning systems can be tricky given all the moving parts. Here are the 4 categories I divide training into with suggestions for each.

1 STRENGTH

- Program as separate element before workout of the day (WOD)
- Balance anterior (push) and posterior (pull), as well as upper and lower, within or between sessions

2 SKILL

- Program as separate element during the week
- Great as a light day, at separate session or as active recovery on days off
- Prior to workout as part of warmup, especially if that skill is used in the WOD

3 STAMINA

- Use before, within, or after the workout
- May reduce soreness when combined with weights
- To really improve, give it a separate day and/or use high-intensity interval training within workouts

4 SUPPLENESS

- Use before, after, and between workouts to enhance mobility and stability
- Consider doing as an entirely different session and/or dedicating your practice its own day

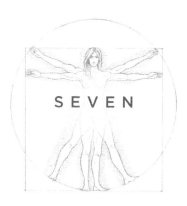

SEVEN

METABOLISM
DISRUPTORS

"Starvation mode," "metabolic damage," "weight loss resistance," and "adrenal fatigue" are all terms you have likely heard related to metabolism and the difficulties people experience with it. However, these terms are a bit controversial, perhaps for good reason, and because of that, we need to explore them before getting into the concept of "metabolic damage."

Let's first start with functional medicine. Functional medicine is a medical specialty that deals with the gray area of dysfunction between health and disease. This is the type of medicine I practice and also where nondiagnostic terms like "adrenal fatigue" and "metabolic damage" come from.

Let me give you a tangible example of this problem. Say you're not feeling so well. You're hungry all the time, urinating more than normal, and gaining weight. When you go to see your traditional doctor, they run your blood sugar to rule out diabetes. If your fasting blood sugar levels are 125, you don't have diabetes, but if they hit 126, you do (diabetes is diagnosed when a fasting blood sugar is 126 or above on two separate occasions). Do you see how utterly ridiculous that is? Long before you get to a fasting blood sugar of 126, you had some serious dysfunction going on. But no one is quite sure what to call it. So medicine calls it a lot of different things, like blood sugar dysregulation, glycemic impairment, prediabetes, and so on. But most of those are not accepted diagnoses. They are simply terms that describe a measurable disturbance that has not yet become a disease.

The terms "metabolic damage," "starvation mode," and others suffer a similar problem. They describe a functional disturbance that may or may not be associated with a particular disease.

Consider this: Long before attention deficit disorder, polycystic ovarian syndrome, fibromyalgia, autism, and chronic fatigue syndrome became diagnoses, they were first called myths and their existence was denied. Meanwhile, forward-thinking docs went right on treating them and defining the characteristics. Saying metabolic damage or starvation mode "is a myth" is a lot like saying prediabetes is a myth. Saying "adrenal fatigue does not exist" is a lot like saying "overtraining doesn't exist." These are functional disturbances that have clinical signs and symptoms that can be picked up on in physical exams and blood labs.

These disturbances may or may not have a corresponding diagnostic label, but that doesn't mean they don't exist. This is the gray area between optimal health and disease, and the area where function starts becoming compromised. This is dysfunction but not yet disease. A person can feel unwell and have metabolic dysfunction without being in an overt disease state. You can have metabolic dysfunction long before you have metabolic disease. Yet, traditional medicine doesn't have many solutions without a firm diagnosis. This is why the field of functional medicine has emerged.

I'm an integrative physician, and I, along with many doctors like me, have been dealing with metabolic damage issues for years. Only we never called it "metabolic damage" or "starvation mode." We called it neuro-endocrine-immune dysfunction. Or we called it by some of its manifestations like "malaise and fatigue." Sometimes when an actual diagnosis could be made, we called it "hypothyroid" or "Hashimoto's thyroiditis."

I have since adopted the term "metabolic damage" because it's more descriptive and easier to comprehend compared to "neuro-endocrine-immune dysfunction." Just remember, the metabolism doesn't "break." In fact, the metabolism is designed to become more rigid. Metabolic compensation and all the manifestations that come along with it are part of its built-in protective mechanism.

LEVELS OF METABOLIC DYSFUNCTION

Let's walk through a hypothetical example that might ring true for you. You decide you want to lose weight and be healthier, so you start a combination of eating less and exercising more. In the beginning, you seem to be doing great. You lose a few pounds right off the bat. So far, so good.

Now you're a week or so in and you start feeling hungry. Your energy falls, and you find yourself craving salty, fatty, sweet foods (in other words, HEC goes out of check). This is a sign the body is starting to move into metabolic compensation. Think of this as metabolic damage level 1.

Because of this compensation, you notice your fat loss slows down. Perhaps it halts altogether. If you're someone with a very pronounced metabolic decline, you may notice you even start gaining weight. And the hunger, energy, and craving issues keep getting worse.

But you're not playing games. You pride yourself on your iron will and rock-solid work ethic. You double your efforts by cutting calories further and ramping up your gym time. Nice. Now you're getting some movement again. Another pound or two down. But it doesn't last. A few weeks later and you're stuck again. This time, the hunger and cravings are worse and your energy is in the toilet. Now you are noticing fragmented sleep and mood issues as well.

Your metabolism is not exactly humming along. Your metabolic rate slows even more. Maybe you try even harder, but now your body just won't budge. You seem to be doing everything "right," but the metabolism digs its heels in. You just moved into metabolic resistance. This is metabolic damage level 2.

You don't get what the hell is going on, but you do know how to deal with it. All you need to do is work harder. You go watch *Conan the Barbarian* and crank up the *Rocky* theme music. You quadruple your effort!

You see very little for your efforts this time. It's been weeks, and you're feeling beat. And now you have other complaints. You start feeling gassy and bloated. The protein shakes you used to tolerate just fine are upsetting your stomach. You're getting heartburn, too. If you're a woman, your menses becomes irregular or disappears. If you're a man, your libido is shot and erections become less predictable.

HEC and SHMEC are further on the downslide. You have this weird feeling of being wired on the inside but tired on the outside. You're starting to feel sick and unwell. You might be anxious, depressed, or both. And now you're slowly gaining weight, looking "waterlogged" despite eating perfectly, and just can't keep up with your workouts anymore. You may even be slowly gaining weight! This is metabolic dysfunction, stage 3 of metabolic damage.

Finally, you feel so unwell you decide to go to the doctor yet again. Several weeks ago, when all these symptoms first started, they ran labs and told you that you were completely normal. Now they see a high TSH, elevated triglycerides, thyroid antibodies, and high fasting blood sugars. They diagnose you with prediabetes and Hashimoto's thyroid (an autoimmune condition of the thyroid that causes low thyroid function). You are officially in metabolic disease, the fourth and final stage of metabolic damage.

Knowing you need some help, you go to a nutrition coach or run-of-the-mill personal trainer. You tell them what's going on, and they say, "You're in starvation mode. You need to eat more and ease up on the exercise." They tell you to double your calorie intake and take it easy on the crazy workout schedule. They in essence take you from an extreme ELEM state into EMEL.

Guess what happens? You blow up like a helium balloon. With your metabolism moving at a snail's pace, *you just did the exact wrong thing.*

You gain about fifteen pounds in six days (which I have seen happen firsthand, by the way)! Of course, it's physiologically impossible to gain that much fat in such a short time, meaning it's almost all water, but still a sign your metabolism is not doing so hot.

You want answers, so you go see a doctor. Maybe they diagnose you with hypothyroid or some other issue. Maybe they say you're normal and nothing is wrong. Obviously, they don't have answers. If you're really unlucky, they tell you to go back to the ELEM approach. But it still won't work and it will just perpetuate the negative cycle and do more damage to your physiology and psyche.

REPAIRING METABOLIC DAMAGE

By now, you've realized you've done everything wrong. But the good news is, you are capable of undoing it.

Stage 1: Metabolic Compensation

How do you know you are in this stage? Hunger, energy, and/or cravings begin to change, and/or weight loss changes or slows.

This phase is easy to deal with. Simply move to any other metabolic toggle. ELEM is not working and the metabolism is too rigid. It is smartest to move to ELEL or EMEM. Both will work. You also may simply need a brief diet break using ESES. Even EMEL will work here provided it's not done for too long. As long as you get off the ELEM train, you'll usually be back on track within a week.

Stage 2: Metabolic Resistance

How do you know you are in this stage? Now sleep and mood start to become noticeably disrupted. Weight loss slows or perhaps you even start gaining weight.

This is also not that hard to deal with, but the approach is slightly different. Just cycle the diet. Spend two to three weeks in ELEL, then change directions toward an EMEM approach. You may also need to take a few other steps including prioritizing rest and recovery, walking, massage, sauna therapy, naps, sex/physical affection, laughter, time with pets, basically anything that lowers stress hormones and restores balance to the neuroendocrine system. Expect to be back on track within one to three months.

Stage 3: Metabolic Dysfunction

How do you know? At this stage, all the other elements of SHMEC start making themselves known, especially other downstream organs from the hypothalamus, the command-and-control center of the metabolism, such as the adrenal, thyroid, and gonads (ovaries and testicles). This is when you start seeing changes in reproductive function. Menses may become irregular, difficult, or absent. Erections may become less responsive and less frequent. Libido in both sexes may decline. This is an especially important barometer of metabolic stress. When the metabolism no longer feels reproductive priorities are essential, you know the stress load is high. Digestive disturbances also often show themselves here with gas and bloating and loose stools or constipation. The digestive tract, often referred to as the "second brain," is a major merging point for the nervous, immune, and endocrine systems. You will also likely begin to see motivation fall and performance and recovery from sport and exercise become more difficult.

At this stage, your best solution is to move into ELEL or ESES. An EMEM approach is too demanding. EMEL will dramatically backfire with weight gain, and ELEM is what got you in this mess in the first place.

Recovering from metabolic dysfunction can take three to twelve months or longer. Recovery depends on how seriously the individual begins to work to reduce the stress by resting more and feeding smartly.

You might wonder why a low-calorie diet such as ESES is the way to go at this point. It all comes down to metabolic potential. Adding a high number of calories into a digestive tract that is no longer responding with adequate digestive secretions and enzyme release is simply asking for trouble. The metabolism needs a break, as does the digestive tract. By moving away from excessive exercise and reducing food to very low-calorie, nutrient-dense foods, the body is able to get enough repair material while not overloading its delicate reserves.

This is also a good time to consider moving to broth-based diets, juices, and smoothies. Just be careful with juicing high-sugar fruits as the body is less tolerable at this point.

Stage 4: Metabolic Disease

How do you know? Simple. Your doctor diagnoses you with a disease.

Once you're here, you have little choice. ELEL is the only option. You'll need to focus all your time on rest and recovery. Walking and a few traditional weight training workouts are likely all you'll be able to do. Consulting with a functional medicine doctor would be smart as well. They'll be able to evaluate thyroid, adrenal, and gonadal function. Supplements, drugs, and hormones may be required. With the right help, you can be back on track within six to eighteen months.

STAGES OF "METABOLIC DAMAGE"

There really is no such thing as "metabolic damage." It's a descriptive term to describe an observable clinical outcome. When diet and exercise are taken to the extreme, individuals may end up somewhere on this spectrum. Most recover just fine; a minority have deeper issues.

ELEL – Eat Less, Exercise Less   **ELEM** – Eat Less, Exercise More
EMEM – Eat More, Exercise More   **EMEL** – Eat More, Exercise Less

1 Metabolic Compensation

- Metabolism adapts
- Boomerang effect
- Increased hunger
- Unpredictable and unstable energy
- Slowed metabolic rate
- Results slow or reverse
- Solution? Switch to another approach besides ELEM

2 Metabolic Resistance

- Person doubles down by eating less and exercising even more
- Hunger, Energy, Cravings (HEC) go further out of check
- Sleep and mood become issues
- Wired (brain) and tired (body)
- Solution? Toggle back and forth between ELEL and EMEM

3 Metabolic Dysfunction

- Person hits wall of fatigue and no motivation
- Depression and/or anxiety
- Digestive issues
- Libido and erection issues
- Body aches and pains
- Tired (brain) and tired (body)
- Solution? ELEL

4 Metabolic Disease

- Person diagnosed with disease
- Most common: hypothyroid, autoimmunity, PCOS, IBS
- Solution? ELEL with specialized diets, medical interventions, and drug treatments

METABOLIC PREHAB: PREPARING THE METABOLISM FOR FAT LOSS

Metabolic rehab and the protocols outlined above are hugely important. But wouldn't it be better to avoid any of these issues in the first place? This is where metabolic "prehab" comes in.

Every spring, you will see it. On the first warm day, hibernating couch potatoes emerge and are seemingly everywhere. They're easy to spot. You can find them jogging in the park, running across the street, laboring down the sidewalk. It's as if they all decided to go out and get in shape all in one day. And if you look closely at their disjointed gait and the agonizing look on their faces, you will see the truth. Because what they are doing is not good for their metabolism. You can't go from a gluttonous couch potato to a CrossFit paleo enthusiast overnight. This is taking the body from one dysfunctional metabolic state (extreme EMEL) to another detrimental metabolic conditioning extreme (ELEM). It's no wonder that by one week into spring, these people are nowhere to be found.

Just as metabolic rehab is about repairing the metabolism after diet abuse, metabolic prehab is about preparing the body to be at its best. Think of it like spring training for the metabolism. Even elite professional athletes don't just jump into their seasons without taking several weeks or months to get the body ready. In order for the metabolism to respond in an efficient, flexible manner to diet and exercise, it needs to be conditioned. This is similar to a warm-up in a workout when you do some mobility and stability work and prepare the body through gentle moving stretches or slow cardio. This same approach should be used with the metabolism as a whole.

So what are we conditioning? The neuro-endocrine-immune system: the brain, the hormones, and the gut (as that is where most of the immune system resides). Poor lifestyle choices make the metabolism less flexible. The command-and-control center of metabolism, the hypothalamus, is an area of the brain that acts like a satellite receiving information from the outside environment as well as the inside cells. It integrates this information and then uses nervous system signals and hormones to adjust the metabolic thermostat.

One of the big pathways in this communication network is the adrenal, thyroid, and gonadal hormonal axis. If the hypothalamus is not receiving or is improperly interpreting the signals it receives, the downstream metabolic effects will also be dysfunctional. Metabolic prehab is all about getting the hypothalamus to respond appropriately. This is done efficiently with three primary tools: walking, contrast hydrotherapy, and adaptogens.

Walking

You already know the benefits to be gained from taking leisurely walks. You don't want to be out of breath. This is not walking for the lungs; this is walking to recalibrate stress hormones as walking lowers cortisol, a major disruptor to optimal hypothalamus function. Walking also dusts the cobwebs off the muscle by amplifying glucose receptors in muscle tissue and decreasing insulin resistance. Slow walking is one of the only forms of movement that simultaneously sensitizes the body to insulin while offering the metabolism relief against cortisol. In metabolic prehab, walking comes first. It also should be ramped up slowly. Start the first week with 5,000 steps a day. The following week, up it to 10,000 steps per day and then move up to 15,000 to 20,000 steps per day. There is no need to go past 20,000 steps per day. Even though it is difficult to overdo walking, it can be done and causes issues for some people. Avoid the temptation to do more. The metabolism works best when you're in the Goldilocks zone: doing not too much, not too little, but just right. For those who are already walking like crazy (such as nurses and others who accumulate huge amounts of daily activity), your goal is to match that excessive activity with relaxing and recovering activities.

Contrast Hydrotherapy

One of the best and most effective approaches for metabolic prehab is contrast hydrotherapy. Contrast hydrotherapy is the alternating use of hot and cold water, and immersion is not necessarily required. In fact, sauna therapy may be as beneficial, if not more so, than water immersion. The real benefit comes from the alternate exposure to hot and cold. The hypothalamus holds the switch on temperature regulation in the body.

If the body gets hot, a host of hormonal and physiological reactions are put in place to cool the body. Sweating ensues, heat shock proteins are released, blood is diverted away from the body's core out to the periphery, thyroid hormone levels change, and immune system alterations are made. When the body is then exposed to cold, blood moves to the core and away from the periphery, different heat shock proteins are activated, metabolic rate jumps, shivering ensues, and brown fat (special fat cells that are more metabolically active and burn more calories) are stimulated.

The back and forth of hot and cold is like exercise for the hypothalamus. It makes it stronger and more flexible. This contrasting treatment also causes whole-body blood changes creating a pumping action. The blood is pushed around the body, perfusing places that need repair and care like joints, the digestive system, muscles, the brain, and the rest of the body.

Perhaps the most important aspect of this treatment is the sweating during hot exposure. POPS (persistent organic pollutants such as chemicals of industry, pesticides, plastics, and other hormone-disrupting chemicals) get stored in fat tissue and are released during fat loss attempts. They then act as irritants to the hypothalamus as well as disruptors of thyroid function. To get rid of toxins, the body eliminates them in breath, urine, feces, and sweat. When it comes to POPS, sweat is likely the most powerful of all modalities. This is why sweating, whether you find it enjoyable or not, is one of the more important aspects of metabolic healing during rehab and metabolic preparation during prehab.

Hot exposure should be three to five times cold exposure to allow for plenty of sweating. Ten to twenty minutes of hot followed by three to four minutes of cold is the typical breakdown I employ with my patients, repeated for three to five rounds. It's best to end on cold unless you will be going to sleep within a few hours. Ending in cold allows the body to exercise the hypothalamus and thyroid to warm you up quickly. Ending in hot causes the body to cool down more quickly given the peripheral dilation of blood vessels near the surface of the skin.

This rapid reduction in body temperature is one of the signals the body uses to induce sleep. Ending in hot is a smart strategy if you're nearing bedtime.

Some may wonder if hot by itself or cold by itself is also acceptable. I have not found cold therapy to be an effective aid by itself except for athletes recovering from exercise. Yes, it does stimulate metabolism, but as you recall, that stimulates hunger. This is why cold therapy has not been shown as an effective fat loss aid. Hot by itself has benefits due to the sweating. If you had to choose an ideal option for metabolic health, a sauna would be a better investment than a hot tub or a cold plunge by itself. Hot tubs use chemicals like bromine and chlorine, which are some of the same chemicals you want your body to detox from and may act as displacers of the important thyroid nutrient iodine. You are far better off sweating in chemical-free heat.

CONTRAST THERAPY

🔥 Hot

- Blood moves from core to periphery
- Sweat increases to cool body
- Heart rate and respiration increase
- Begins relaxing (parasympathetic)
- Turns stimulating (sympathetic)
- Stimulates cellular repair proteins
- Thyroid increases (TBG release of T4)

❄️ Cold

- Blood moves from periphery to core
- Shivering ensues to warm body
- Heart rate and respiration decrease
- Starts stimulating (sympathetic)
- Turns relaxing (parasympathetic)
- Stimulates cellular repair proteins
- Thyroid may increase (increase TRH)

How To:

1. Hot 15 min
2. Cold 1–3 min
3. Repeat 3–5 rounds
4. End in cold

Benefits:

- Exercise for the hypothalamic-pituitary axes (especially the thyroid)
- Relaxing, restorative, and regenerative
- Same physiological effects of light exercise

- Lowers blood pressure post-treatment
- May lower stress hormones post-treatment
- May reduce cardiovascular risk with repeated use

Additional Prep

In addition to walking and contrast hot-and-cold therapy, there are several other elements to metabolic prehab. You also want to get the digestive system and the mitochondria (the energy-producing organelles in every cell) ready. If the hypothalamus is the command-and-control center of the metabolism, the gut is the five-star general. The gut is a hub of metabolic activity and the most important crossroads of the nervous, endocrine, and immune systems. The gut also contains the most fascinating area of study currently in metabolism research: the microbiome. In order to understand the prehab for the gut, let's briefly walk through how this system works.

From the time you see, smell, or think about food, your body starts to engage a host of nervous system and hormonal activity designed to digest, absorb, and assimilate the fuel and nutrients your body needs.

Once you start chewing the food, your brain and mouth start to communicate in what is often called the neurolingual response and the cephalic phase response. Basically, this means as you chew and taste your food, the nervous system in the mouth sends information to the brain about the tastes, textures, and flavors that may be coming. Sweetness represents carbohydrates; meaty, chewy, and savory represent protein. Then there is creamy, chewy, cakey, sour, and a whole host of other textures, flavors, and tastes. These attributes signal the brain, which then signals other organs like the stomach, the pancreas, and the small intestines to get to work secreting certain enzymes and other factors to break down the coming food constituents.

The stomach releases hydrochloric acid to aid protein breakdown and other signaling molecules like CCK and ghrelin that signal hunger reduction or elevation, respectively. When the food is acidic enough, it passes into the upper small intestines and the gallbladder releases bile salts while the pancreatic duct drops in amylase, protease, trypsin, chymotrypsin, and lipase. All these enzymes are designed to break down the food further while the bile helps to emulsify the fat you have consumed. At the same time, cells lining the gut wall continue to sample the food passing by. They then send signals to the brain to control hunger. These compounds are called incretins and include hormones like GIP and GLP. Lower down the digestive tract, there are other incretins like PYY. These compounds are heavily involved in hunger suppression. Protein and sticky viscous fibers signal these cells to slow down digestion and reduce hunger. If you have ever made a pot of oatmeal and watched the thick viscous layer stick to the side of the bowl, you have an idea how food like this might stick to the walls of the digestive tract signaling long-term fullness. This is why soluble fiber and protein are shown to be so appetite suppressing.

From there, small food particles such as sugars/starches (monosaccharides, disaccharides, polysaccharides, etc.), protein (amino acids), and fats (saturated and unsaturated) all begin to get absorbed.

The better the upper digestive process went, the more efficiently these food elements can be absorbed and processed. When the food is less digested, it is more likely to trigger negative reactions in the digestive tract.

The next step is for the microbiome to get to work. As food passes into the lower small intestines and colon, bacteria go to work on it. These bacteria are often called probiotics and make up what scientists now refer to as the microbiome. There are more bacteria living in your gut than there are cells in your body. Even though the digestive tract is technically outside of the body, because it is basically one continuous hollow tube from mouth to anus, some scientists call the microbiome the largest organ in the body. These bacteria get fed from the foods we don't digest and absorb. Fiber seems to be especially beneficial in feeding the good bacteria in the gut.

The critical thing to understand about the microbiome is that we each appear to have our own bacterial makeup, almost like a fingerprint. These bacteria digest food particles we did not and in the process generate all kinds of useful by-products including vitamins and minerals like butyrate, which feeds the cells lining the digestive tract, vitamin K, and many of the B vitamins. These digestive "bugs" also release many bioactive compounds as they undergo their own metabolism. Some of these compounds are highly beneficial, sending healthy metabolic signals helpful to immune function and metabolic health. Other bacteria send disruptive bioactive compounds into the body that can trigger immunoreactivity and potentially play a role in autoimmunity.

The research in this area is extremely robust. However, we still don't have a full understanding of how to take advantage of the microbiome in the way we would like to. The current understanding regarding the microbiome is that microbial diversity may be more important than the amount or types of bacteria present.

The other thing to know is that the microbiome is extremely responsive to changes in diet, including the type and amounts of food consumed. This is one explanation for why sudden changes in diet can result in uncomfortable digestive reactions like loose stool, gas, bloating, pain, and cramping. These symptoms are a sure sign the microbiome is adjusting and reacting to dietary habits. Constipation, loose stool, and gas and bloating are not normal metabolic states, and their presence is a very important consideration in your evaluation of SHMEC. Remember, SHMEC is not just about sleep, hunger, mood, energy, and cravings. The term is meant to be a catchall phrase for all metabolic biofeedback. The digestive system and the microbiome are a huge hub of metabolic activity and the crossroads between the immune, hormone, and nervous systems.

When you eat, the microbiome blooms; when you don't, it shrinks. When healthy bacteria are dominating in the gut, they secrete beneficial compounds and ensure the protective mucosal layer of the digestive system is hardy and functional. This means fewer immune reactions, less gut irritation, and more beneficial and synergistic metabolic activity (such as vitamin production by the bacteria). There are certain nutrients that seem to bolster this process, glutamine being chief among them. Glutamine is an amino acid that acts as a preferred substrate for the cells lining the intestines. It also is released in times of stress as it is also a foundational metabolite in healthy immune responses.

At the same time, when you eat lots of refined sugars and starches, you may be pushing less favorable bacteria to propagate in the digestive tract. These bacteria, known as gram-negative, shed a compound called LPS (lipopolysaccharide), which is extremely detrimental. LPS is known as endotoxin and causes the immune system to react strongly whenever it is around in large numbers. Although sugar/starch may increase the types and amounts of gram-negative bacteria, the presence of fat makes matters worse. LPS is lipophilic, meaning it likes fat and is fat soluble.

LPS hitches a ride into the body by incorporating into fat that we then absorb. This triggers strong inflammatory reactions. If you have ever had a pizza, burger, and/or alcohol binge and woke up achy, stiff, and in pain, you may have experienced this LPS reaction on the immune system. This may also explain some of the negative effects of high-fat diets like keto. Imagine a person eating the standard Western junk food diet made up of over 50 percent starch and sugar, then switching to a high-fat diet. They would have a ton of LPS as a result of a consistent overgrowth of gram-negative bacteria. When they switch to a higher fat diet, they may be getting large doses of LPS into the system. This may be one of the reasons some individuals struggle with a flu-like feeling after starting a keto diet, known as the keto flu.

ELEL AND THE GUT

Prehab is where the ELEL approach to living shines even brighter. Reducing calories to very low levels is far less possible with lots of exercise, as exercise both uses fuel and micronutrients *and* causes increased hunger for highly palatable foods rich in starch, sugar, salt, and fat. Those are the very foods that can cause dysbiosis or unfavorable bacterial growth. Think about what that means. Fewer nutrients are coming in due to decreased calorie and nutrient intake. That then is followed by binges of foods rich in calories but devoid of healthy vitamins and minerals. Those same foods both increase negative bacterial propagation and translocate LPS into the bloodstream. Add to that exercise, which makes for greater hunger, further pushes nutrient use, and causes more cravings for many. The result is a person who is extremely tired and metabolically stressed, with aches, stiffness, and increased susceptibility to infections and inflammatory diseases, especially autoimmune.

ELEL reduces calories without the extra exercise but rather with a focus on walking instead.

This reduces cravings and hunger, allowing the GI system to process more nutrient-dense food but less food overall, giving it a rest from constantly being bombarded with the need to digest and assimilate. Resting the GI system is critical for getting it optimal once more. From there, clinically, I add a good digestive enzyme (I prefer one with HCL), glutamine (ten to twenty grams daily for a few weeks to a few months), and a full-spectrum spore-based probiotic.

Spore-based probiotic supplementation has been shown to enhance the protective layer of the gut. These bacteria may also be the only kind that actually survive the digestive process and are able to have more impact on gut function and gut health. These spore-based probiotics have been a huge part of the human diet since the dawn of man. It was impossible not to consume some of the soil on the food we hunted and gathered. That soil contained the very same spore-based probiotics that became synergistic commensals with us humans.

By giving the gut a break with ELEL as well as adding digestive aids (enzymes), digestive healers (glutamine), and digestive health promoters (spore-based probiotics), we prepare and prime it for optimal digestion absorption and assimilation. Our guts can be a steaming cauldron of inflammatory potential or a calming, soothing functional bastion of quality health inputs.

The final step of metabolic rehab has to do with the energy factories of our cells, the mitochondria. If your cell was a city, the mitochondria would be its power plants. These mitochondria have a series of membranes that control the biochemistry of energy production by creating energy gradients that build up charge. These gradients create the power to produce ATP, which the cell uses to power itself.

The issue occurs when the mitochondria are constantly overloaded by excess energy. This is one of the fundamental reasons why overconsuming calories is so detrimental to metabolic function.

When your body breaks down macronutrients like fat and sugar, the common biochemical product is acetyl-CoA. This compound then is used by the mitochondria to begin energy production. Now imagine you were working on a coal plant and kept feeding coal into the fires at a faster rate than it could be burned. What would happen? You would likely snuff out the fires due to lack of oxygen, make the power plant far less efficient, and do damage to the machinery. The same happens to the mitochondria.

The mitochondria make up a highly active place and generate plenty of free radicals. If the flow of acetyl-CoA is slow and steady, the mitochondria easily handle things and continue humming along. If the mitochondria become overwhelmed through consistent overeating and too much acetyl-CoA, their function falters and they begin spewing more and more free radicals (let's call it metabolic smoke). A free radical is an active molecule that is searching for electrons and will whip around the mitochondrial membranes, ripping apart cellular machinery. The mitochondria and cell have their own antioxidant protections that catch these hot radicals and put the fire out. But the harder the mitochondria have to work, the more free radicals escape and do damage.

This then causes a bottom-up issue where energy production at the cellular level is compromised. Fatigue, faltering motivation, aches and pains, and every other conceivable issue starts to manifest. Hormones are also contingent on mitochondrial function, and poor mitochondrial health also leads to dysfunctional hormone production.

Again, the ELEL approach works wonders here. The very low-calorie diet without a ton of exercise, but rather mostly walking, allows the mitochondria to repair and recharge. Walking is a wonderful and gentle first step to conditioning the mitochondria for future, more-intense exercise.

To help the mitochondria, the prehab process involves eating a low-calorie, nutrient-dense diet while also providing the building blocks of mitochondrial membranes. This is where essential fats like fish oil come in. This is also where protein intake is important. The antioxidants used to protect mitochondria come from amino acids, which come from dietary protein. One protein in particular has been shown to enhance mitochondrial glutathione stores above all others: whey protein. Add long periods of fasting to this prehab regime and you give the mitochondria everything it needs to heal. Fasting twelve to twenty hours daily ramps up autophagy (the longer the fast the better). Autophagy is the cells' natural self-healing, recycling, and regenerating procedure. When food is not available, the cell has time to go seek out and clean up damaged cell membranes and cellular debris. Add walking, which exercises the mitochondria, getting them prepared and flexible, then add adequate protein to ensure cellular antioxidant defenses. Fish oils and other essential fats and phospholipids provide the building blocks required for high-charged efficient mitochondria to be rebuilt.

STEP-BY-STEP PREHAB

Now that you know why prehab matters, here is how to do it. Four weeks prior to beginning any diet (ELEM or EMEM), move to an ELEL approach with at least twelve to sixteen hours of complete fasting. Walk 10,000 to 20,000 steps daily. Drink four to eight liters of pure mineral water daily. Sleep seven to nine hours daily and/or nap to reach this total sleep time.

Supplement with adaptogens. Adaptogens are plants that have been shown in research to raise or lower metabolic function based on need. They help you adapt to overwork, stress, and strain. Rhodiola and ashwagandha are my favorites and have the best evidence base. Rhodiola is mostly for fatigue and depression when both the body and the brain are tired. Ashwagandha is for fatigue and anxiety, when you're tired in the body but wired in the brain, which often causes insomnia. Another of my favorite adaptogens is not always thought of as an adaptogen, CBD.

The endocannabinoid system influences every metabolic action you can think of and is often a great approach to use to help the hypothalamus and all its downstream targets. The typical doses for rhodiola and ashwagandha are 200–600 mg and 600–1,200 mg of standardized products, respectively (rhodiola standardized to rosavin and salidroside and ashwagandha to withanolides).

Add in contrast hydrotherapy. Hot tub to cold shower will work, but access to a sauna and cold plunge is even better. Shoot for three to five rounds of ten to twenty minutes hot followed by one to three minutes cold. End on cold unless it is evening and you will be sleeping soon.

Take a full-spectrum digestive enzyme daily (look for HCL, protease, lipase, amylase, trypsin, chymotrypsin, etc.). Use L-glutamine powder, consuming 10–20 grams daily during metabolic prehab. A spore-based probiotic is also a consideration. Although the science on probiotic intake is far from satisfactory, the existing evidence and my clinical experience suggest it as a powerful metabolic primer.

Finally, for mitochondrial health, a good quality fish oil supplying between 500 mg and 1,000 mg of EPA and DHA is useful. If you can tolerate dairy, an additional 20–40 grams of whey protein one to two times daily is one of the best and tastiest approaches to bolstering antioxidant production in the body. Although many people are overly reliant on antioxidant intake from food, this pales in comparison to what the body makes. Your best bet for antioxidant protection comes from enticing your body to produce more.

One final bonus consideration for metabolic prehab is nutrient supplementation through the use of what I call a metabolic multivitamin. This is a special multiple vitamin and mineral supplement that provides the body with extra nutritive insurance during an ELEL prehab process.

These vitamin supplements use the active forms of the B vitamins such as methyl folate and riboflavin-5-phosphate as well as magnesium, zinc, and selenium. In addition, and perhaps more importantly, the use of activators, antioxidants, and detox aids to support mitochondrial function and repair is critical for some. The triple cocktail of CoQ10 (100–200 mg), acetyl-L-carnitine (1,000 mg), and alpha lipoic acid (200–400 mg) is a powerful formula to restore mitochondrial function.

METABOLIC PREHAB

Spending time conditioning the metabolism prior to weight loss attempts can help control hunger and cravings and speed results. Think of this like "spring training" for the metabolism.

Biorhythms
The command and control center of the metabolism and the center of the stress thermostat. Reduce stress on this system, and you aid function to the thyroid, adrenals, and gonads.

Biome
A central hub of metabolic processing. The functional crossroads of the neuroendocrine immune system. Focus here to decrease inflammation and prime metabolic processing.

Biochemistry
The body requires adequate nutrient availability and processing. This means giving the body nutritional elements that power cellular machinery as well as ensuring appropriate hormonal action, signaling, and sensitivity.

Bioenergetics
The energy factories of the cell. Responsible for burning fat and other fuel for energy. Support here reduces "metabolic smoke" (free radical) and increases metabolic flexibility.

Biorhythms
- Walk 10K steps daily
- Sleep 8 hours daily
- Wake at same time each morning
- Early daylight exposure
- Contrast hydrotherapy
- Mobility practice (i.e., melt, gentle yoga, etc.)
- Adaptogen use

Biome
- Include fermented foods in the diet
- Increase fiber intake
- Probiotics, prebiotics and postbiotics MAY be useful based on evidence associated with particular conditions or complaints

Biochemistry
- Supplement with a multivitamin
- Restore insulin sensitivity
- Lower cortisol
- Lower meal size
- Decrease meal frequency
- Fasting may have benefit

Bioenergetics
- Alpha-lipoic acid 200mg
- Acetyl-L-carnitine 1000mg
- CoQ10 100mg
- Whey protein to increase glutathione and antioxidant capacity
- Supplementation with essential fats and phospholipids for cell membrane health

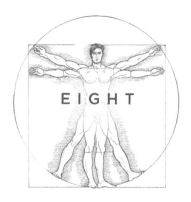

THE METABOLIC
PHYSIOLOGIST

nderstanding the differences between each person's unique metabolism is like trying to make out the characteristics of a person who's hundreds of yards away. If you saw me walking toward you from that distance, even if you had to squint, you would be able to deduce that I am a human. There'd be no mistaking me for a dog or a giraffe. For one thing, I'd be walking on two legs. For another, I'm a pretty big guy, so you might not even have to squint. Then, as I started moving closer to you, you'd be able to see that I am male. By the time I got even closer, you'd see that I am bald. As I started talking, you'd notice my funny accent. The closer I get to you, the more you can see what makes me unique.

At the surface level, there doesn't seem to be a significant difference between male and female metabolism. Not until we look closer do we see what distinguishes them from one another, and the closer you look, the more you see.

The biggest difference is the specific sources of stress the metabolism is on the lookout for. Men and women have different physiological drivers dictating their priorities. Men are looking out into the world and determining two things: (1) Is it safe? and (2) Who can I have sex with? Women, on the other hand, are asking: (1) Is it safe? and (2) Who would make a good baby with me? In other words, men are looking to spread their seeds while women are looking for the best genes.

Females are the gender of childbearing, and that reality demands the metabolism be a little more sensitive and refined. This is why women can have more negative reactions to stress, especially at certain times of their menstrual cycles. When it senses a baby could be coming along, the metabolism becomes hypervigilant to create the safest, best environment for the new addition.

From the time they hit puberty, women start understanding how these changes are directly impacting their entire physiology and causing potentially massive fluctuations in HEC and SHMEC.

Men, however, remain pretty static hormonally speaking. Women also have more stages of life they have to transition through hormonally. Whereas women go through puberty, pregnancy, perimenopause, menopause, and postmenopause, men go through only puberty and andropause. These changes in hormones are one of the reasons why women tend to find that one way of dieting or exercising might work at one stage of their life but not at another. Similarly, one thing might work really well during the first half of their menstrual cycle but not during the second. The sex hormones are impacting their metabolic stress barometer, so figuring out what works best and when can take time for women.

HORMONE HIERARCHY

When most people think about hormones, testosterone, estrogen, and progesterone are the first that come to mind. However, when it comes to metabolism, sex steroids are not the primary players. In fact, their role is somewhat secondary. According to the hierarchy of hormonal influence on metabolism:

- The base of the pyramid is calories.
- Next comes insulin and cortisol.
- Third comes the thyroid and adrenal hormones.
- *Last* come estrogen, progesterone, and testosterone at the peak.

Therefore, although sex hormones are capable of influencing the other, more impactful hormones, they are not as important as many think.

On the other hand, insulin (a hormone that regulates food uptake and storage in cells) and cortisol (a hormone that regulates adaptations to stress) are capable of wildly disrupting metabolism. Think of insulin and cortisol as two rambunctious kids on a seesaw. Imbalances in one negatively influence the other. Sex steroids, like estrogen, progesterone, and testosterone, play a moderating role, convincing them to slow down and play nicely. They are not running the show but definitely impacting the behavior of the key players.

Another common misconception is that receptors for sex steroids are located only in the breast, uterus, ovaries, or testicles, when in fact they are all over the body. They can be found in the brain, muscle tissue, and fat tissue. And these hormones don't just impact reproduction—each one can have a subtle influence over everything else and in doing so, have a significant impact on HEC and SHMEC.

ESTROGEN AND PROGESTERONE

The best way to conceptualize the action of estrogen and progesterone is to picture nonidentical twin sisters. They are twins because estrogen and progesterone are completely reliant on each other but serve different purposes. Progesterone helps the body hear estrogen (by priming the estrogen receptor), and estrogen helps the body respond to progesterone (by also priming its receptor). Because of this, these two hormones do not like being without each other, and their codependence becomes most noticeable during periods that disrupt one or the other (e.g., during periods of stress and at perimenopause when progesterone falls). These "sisters" don't do well when either is out of balance or if one's influence is absent altogether.

Let's look at what happens with these sisters throughout the menstrual cycle. In the first half, from the first day of bleeding to ovulation fourteen days later, estrogen is dominating. She is very driven, adventurous, and rambunctious. She wants to go and attack life.

Estrogen keeps both insulin and cortisol at bay. She's more stress resistant and can tolerate higher amounts of calories and exercise. Estrogen is more entrepreneurial and athletic than her sister; she resembles testosterone—the brother of the two sisters—in this way. When estrogen is around, EMEM is the ideal toggle. Estrogen helps metabolism multitask better. In the estrogen state, women are able to better achieve simultaneous fat loss and muscle gain due to its moderating influence on insulin sensitivity. Estrogen makes the female body more sensitive to insulin, meaning a woman in a low-calorie state will burn less muscle and more fat. It also means a woman who finds herself in calorie excess will be more likely to store some of the calories as muscle as opposed to fat. Estrogen also acts as a shield against the stress hormone cortisol, allowing her to tolerate greater amounts of stress with fewer negative effects. Although training and eating like an athlete (i.e., being in EMEM) is ideal when estrogen is dominating, it also makes women less reactive and more responsive to the normally more stressful metabolic toggles of ELEM and EMEL. Estrogen also raises the brain chemicals serotonin and dopamine, which makes women feel more at ease, more confident, more driven and ambitious, and more likely to take risks.

Compared to her sister, progesterone is more of a homebody. If estrogen loves interval training, weights, and CrossFit, progesterone is more into relaxing, meditation, and walks in the garden. She wants to read books and do yoga. She also tends to worry—*a lot.* She's worried about the world, she's worried about her sister, she's worried about having a baby, and she's worried about being safe.

Progesterone behaves the opposite of estrogen when it comes to insulin. She makes the female metabolism more insulin resistant.

However, the two sisters work together when it comes to cortisol. Progesterone helps estrogen manage cortisol in a healthy manner.

Progesterone also regulates the number one relaxing brain chemical, GABA. This is why she is needed to calm her rambunctious sister down.

When estrogen is running around like crazy without progesterone, she's going to get in trouble. It's also not much fun when uptight progesterone is running the show, which she rarely does. The two have to have each other's backs. Estrogen forces progesterone out of her introverted shell, and progesterone reminds estrogen to be careful and look before she leaps. The two together are what keeps things balanced and running smoothly.

During the second half of the menstrual cycle, things get a little more interesting. The first half of the menstrual cycle is all about estrogen. She is playing by herself while progesterone is at home napping. In fact, the first two weeks of the menstrual cycle, prior to ovulation, progesterone levels in women resemble progesterone levels in men. It is not until after ovulation that progesterone "wakes up" and comes out to play with her sister.

This is where things can get a little complicated as there are two ways to look at the menstrual cycle post-ovulation. From a relative perspective (meaning estrogen levels relative to progesterone levels), progesterone is dominant. But from an absolute perspective, estrogen levels are still pretty high.

To make this clearer, let's divide the menstrual cycle into four phases instead of just two. Phase 1 is the week of menses. At this point, estrogen is waking up while progesterone is asleep. This is called the early follicular phase. The follicle, which contains the egg, begins to mature for the next attempt at reproduction.

Week 2 sees estrogen really ramp up her activity. The follicle ripens and prepares to release the egg. This is late follicular phase.

Now there is a surge in luteinizing hormone and this signals the egg to release. This is the middle of the cycle, ovulation. Right around this time, you see a brief rise in testosterone, and sometimes a small dip in estrogen, which is part of the reason some women will spot bleed during this time. Testosterone's influence causes women to be more sexually proactive.

The follicle becomes the corpus luteum, which is the source of progesterone. This is phase 3 or the early luteal phase and sees estrogen and progesterone playing together. This time of the cycle can act as a key source of biofeedback for women. If progesterone does not adequately wake up, a female can find herself remaining in an estrogen-dominant state at a time when she should be moderating things for potential fertilization of the egg. If progesterone fails to make herself known, women can begin to see mood changes, irritability, and an ever-increasing feeling of illness and premenstrual difficulty until menses arrives and resets the cycle.

Phase 4 is the late luteal phase. This is the premenstrual period when estrogen and progesterone both begin to fall, get tired, and want to go to sleep. At this time, there can be an "unmasking of testosterone." Since the sisters are in bed, the brother's influence can be seen more and sometimes female libido will jump once more in and around menses.

Now you can see two ways to look at the menstrual cycle: a follicular phase when estrogen dominates and a luteal phase when progesterone dominates, or a menstrual time with lower levels of estrogen premenstrually and menstrually and an ovulatory time with higher levels of estrogen the week before and after ovulation.

When estrogen and progesterone are both present, progesterone is usually exerting a moderating influence. Biochemically, progesterone is making the body more insulin resistant and stress aware.

METABOLISM AND MENSES: OPTION 1

Cycling diet and exercise with the menstrual cycle

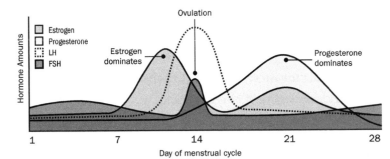

Day 1 (menses starts) ✗

Day 2–7 (early follicular phase)

Day 8–14 (late follicular phase)

- Follicle develops
- Estrogen rising
- Progesterone low
- More insulin sensitive
- Less stress reactive

S	M	T	W	T	F	S
1	2	✗3	4	5	6	7
8	9	10	11	12	13	14
15	16	17✓	18	19	20	21
22	23	24	25	26	27	28
29	30	31				

Eat More, Exercise More (EMEM)

- More frequent workouts
- Plenty of weight-training
- More cardio, HIIT, and metcons
- More calories and carbs to fuel training

Day 14 (ovulation) ✓

Day 15–21 (early luteal phase)

Day 22–28 (late luteal phase)

- Corpus luteum forms
- Progesterone higher
- Less relative estrogen
- More insulin resistant
- More stress reactive

Eat Less, Exercise Less (ELEL)

- More walking and less exercise
- More weights and less cardio
- Relax, recover, restore
- Manage stress as a priority

METABOLISM AND MENSES: OPTION 2

Cycling diet and exercise with the menstrual cycle

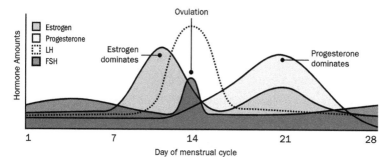

Day 22–28 (late luteal phase)
Day 1 (menses starts) ✗
Day 2–7 (early follicular phase)

- Follicle develops
- Estrogen rising
- Progesterone low
- More insulin sensitive
- Less stress reactive

Day 8–14 (late follicular phase)
Day 14 (ovulation) ✔
Day 15–21 (early luteal phase)

- Corpus luteum forms
- Progesterone higher
- Less relative estrogen
- More insulin resistant
- More stress reactive

S	M	T	W	T	F	S
1	2	✗3	4	5	6	7
8	9	10	11	12	13	14
15	16	17✔	18	19	20	21
22	23	24	25	26	27	28
29	30	31				

Eat More, Exercise More (EMEM)
More frequent workouts
Plenty of weight-training
More cardio, HIIT, and metcons
More calories and carbs to fuel training

Eat Less, Exercise Less (ELEL)
More walking and less exercise
More weights and less cardio
Relax, recover, restore
Manage stress as a priority

Now is the time for meditative yoga, long walks, reading, and cuddling with your sexual partner. This is also an ideal time for ELEL, when women are more relaxed and less motivated to do any intense training.

If the egg that was released does not get fertilized, estrogen and progesterone fall off abruptly, and with both gone, there are resulting changes to HEC and SHMEC. During this time, it helps to do everything you can to balance HEC and SHMEC while paying particular attention to the mood element. Estrogen and progesterone have a great effect on brain chemicals like dopamine, serotonin, and GABA. The combination of these brain chemicals gives a focused, relaxed, content state of mind. When estrogen and progesterone fall at menses, the mental state can feel exactly the opposite.

A useful trick here is to mimic some of the mood-balancing impacts of estrogen and progesterone with cocoa powder. Cocoa powder is cocoa beans that have been roasted and pulverized, and some of the compounds found within it act as brain chemical mimickers. Phenylethylamine (PEA) is a dopamine mimicker. Cocoa contains serotonin and anandamide, which relaxes like GABA. Cocoa powder, however, doesn't have all the fat and extra calories that chocolate has. You can put two tablespoons of cocoa powder in water and drink it like coffee. In fact, adding cocoa to coffee has been shown to amplify the energizing impact of coffee while decreasing its anxiety-producing impact. You can even add a bit of non-calorie sweetener. Even though the bitter taste of plain cocoa is most ideal, a little sweet may be preferred by some. Just make sure it does not trigger cravings for more sweet.

TESTOSTERONE

Most people know testosterone is tied to libido in both men and women, but they don't know it's also linked to ambition and drive.

If I have a client whom I suspect is having an issue with testosterone, I'm less interested in the frequency of his erections than I am the quality of his brain. If he's feeling down, lethargic, not driven, or not at all ambitious, a testosterone issue is my first suspect. Testosterone is the "I want to win" hormone that drives the male ego and makes many of us so competitive. Testosterone also gives men more chiseled lines, sharper jaws, even larger penises (intrauterine testosterone exposure may be a prime determinant of penis size), all of which women tend to be attracted to, especially during certain points of their menstrual cycles when estrogen is high. Interestingly, when estrogen is low as they get closer to menses, women tend to prefer more estrogen-dominant men. The first kind of man is the one they want to reproduce with but who they also know is likely to want to spread his seed everywhere, whereas the second man is the one they think will be more likely to stay home and help them care for the baby.

Testosterone can have both similar and different impacts on women. Women who have had testosterone therapy might see clitoral enlargement, more chiseled jawlines, or voice box changes.

There is one major difference, however, between the influence of testosterone on male and female physiques. In men, testosterone tends to be associated with leaner waistlines and more firm muscular physiques. In women, higher testosterone may actually thicken the waistline. This highlights the waist-slimming potential of estrogen over testosterone. Women already have the best belly-burning hormonal makeup in estrogen and progesterone.

You can see this in women who become highly active in intense sports conditioning and metabolic conditioning programs like CrossFit. These forms of activity generate large amounts of testosterone and human growth hormone (HGH), resulting in more pronounced muscles, leaner bodies, thicker waists, and less pronounced hourglass shapes.

PREGNANCY AND MENOPAUSE

Progesterone dominates pregnancy when women essentially remain in the luteal phase of the menstrual cycle that occurs after ovulation and before menses. From fertilization through the time they stop breastfeeding, progesterone levels are high. It's hard to lose weight during this time because the metabolism is convinced you need fat on your body to continue to support the baby.

During perimenopause, if you don't ovulate, you don't get progesterone. It's as if progesterone is sick and wants to stay in bed. Then estrogen starts to miss her sister and becomes volatile, bouncing high to low and jumping all over the place. One minute, the woman will feel fine, and the next, she's extremely irritated. She might get hot flashes. It feels like she's all over the place, but the good news is, there are some things she can do to get everything under control. Remember that progesterone is the caretaker. She's all about managing stress reactions and convincing women to avoid overdoing it. When she's gone, women need to become their own caretakers. They need to mother and nurture themselves, which is oftentimes tough for women who are always taking care of everyone else. In my experience working with women at this stage, the hardest thing is simply convincing them to stop expending so much energy toward others and start focusing on themselves. Now is not the time for dieting and intense training. Instead, it's ideal to move toward mindfulness and meditation (and in the next chapter, I'll walk you through exactly how to do that). They also might consider talking to their doctors about oral progesterone therapies. Regardless of how you opt to handle it, this is not the time to be the CrossFit, paleo person. It's time for calm, quiet, and comfort.

As a woman enters menopause, estrogen falls off as well, and by the time she's in postmenopause, testosterone levels can become relatively more dominant, though it still remains low.

Some women are even given testosterone therapy at this point, because testosterone can be made into estrogen. At this time, some women also start looking more like men, with expanding waists and less defined features. But don't stress, ladies—this change goes both ways. Men also start looking more female as they age and become more estrogen dominant, which is why you see some eighty-year-old couples and can't tell who's who.

HORMONES IN MEN

In men, testosterone is constantly battling with insulin and cortisol, meaning a man who is not exercising his body in some way will eventually and inevitably become dominated by stress. These are the men who turn into the stereotypical fat businessman who can't get an erection. To keep their testosterone at healthy levels, men need to engage in workouts that leave their muscles burning, such as weight lifting. Most people assume they're only getting the maximum benefit from a workout if they're breathless, but for men, having that burn in their muscles matters more.

Men also can experience lower testosterone levels when they have a drop of any major macronutrient, such as carbohydrates and protein, or some micronutrients, particularly zinc, magnesium, and vitamin D. Think about early man who was outside all day finding quality nutrition, getting plenty of micronutrients from the sun, and filling up on his latest kill at the end of the day. If he didn't have adequate nutrition, the last thing he'd care about would be having sex. This is why extreme low-carb or low-fat diets often leave men lacking libido.

During andropause, or male menopause, testosterone begins to drop dramatically. During this phase, it becomes crucial that men put real time and effort into moving and weight training. It's time to pick up the pace and help your body produce as much testosterone as possible.

THE UPS AND DOWNS OF ERECTIONS

Guys in your thirties or forties, see if this sounds familiar: You consider yourself pretty healthy. You do pretty much the right things when it comes to training and diet. But lately, that doesn't seem to be enough. These days, you've been feeling fatigued, maybe even unmotivated, and you're noticing your pants are getting a bit snug around your middle. Maybe that chest you've worked to keep nice and tight is getting a little soft. But what's bothering you the most, because, let's face it, it's the biggest concern of them all, is your erections—more specifically, your inability to rely on them showing up or sustaining them when they do.

If this is ringing a bell, don't despair. You are not alone, and I have had the clients to prove it. Because although it might seem straightforward, there is more to the male erection than meets the eye.

An erection is a closely orchestrated event between the nervous system and blood flow into and out of the penis. When the brain registers a "sexually relevant" cue, nerve impulses are sent to the penis. This triggers a host of biochemical events that involve chemicals like nitric oxide (NO) being released, which then trigger cellular cyclic GMP, which open the blood vessels allowing more blood to flow in. While blood flow is increased going in, a spongy layer of the penis, rich with capillaries, becomes engorged, causing pressure to build up. This hydrostatic pressure causes it to inflate.

This is all also contingent on a separate set of blood vessels that drain the penis. These vessels start to constrict under the increasing pressure and other biochemical events. The coordinated action of the incoming blood vessels, and the building pressure, is what allows blood to rush in and stay in, creating an erection.

The Three Bs

When you think of testosterone, libido, and erections, you have to consider the three Bs: brain, biochemistry, and blood flow.

Brain

The sexual brain can be thought of as containing both stimulators and repressors. Emily Nagoski, PhD, author of *Come as You Are*, calls these accelerators and brakes. In order for sexual desire to occur and sexual arousal to engage, the accelerators need to be turned up while the brakes are turned down. For example, say you're hard at work trying to meet a seemingly unmeetable deadline. Your girlfriend passes by and stops to give you a quick shoulder massage (aka the stimulator). Your brain registers this and hits the accelerator, but before anything can happen, your brain reminds you of all the work stress you're dealing with.

It works like this: You're sitting on the couch working frantically to get a proposal done for work. You're stressed. Your girlfriend sits down next to you and starts rubbing on you. You register a "sexually relevant stimulus." This hits the accelerators, but when the brain checks in on the context, all that stress slams on the brakes. The degree to which the stimulus can amplify the accelerators, combined with the degree to which the stress is stepping on the brakes, will determine the quality of the erection and response (in case you're wondering, this is exactly why foreplay and context are so much more important for sexual desire, arousal, and function in women). So if you've ever found yourself in a situation where you have a strong sexual desire but aren't able to perform, just remember it is that common, it does happen to every guy, and it isn't a big deal.

To understand this brain effect better, think "point and shoot." The two branches of the nervous system are P, parasympathetic, and S, sympathetic. Parasympathetic is relaxing and sympathetic is stimulating. The balance of P and S is critical.

To get a boner, you need adequate P, or parasympathetic outflow. Think P for "point" to remember this. To ejaculate requires adequate sympathetic outflow. Think S for "shoot." A man who ejaculates too quickly and/or has weak erections is dealing with poor parasympathetic (relaxing) outflow. Many things can cause this: being overworked, being overwhelmed, alcohol, stress, mood medications, or any condition that disrupts nerve signaling such as diabetes.

A man who's unable to ejaculate or takes forever to ejaculate may be suffering from the opposite: poor sympathetic outflow. This too can be caused by stress, mood medications, and diabetes. This may also be a sign of the use of Viagra or another PDE5 inhibitor. For younger men who aren't overweight, this is almost always a result of some type of stress effect or medication.

Another brain concern has to do with the command-and-control center of the metabolism. The hypothalamus is an area of the brain that receives signals from other hormones and then coordinates other hormone-producing organs in the body. The hypothalamus registers all the signals from the environment (sight, sound, temperature, etc.) and signals from inside the body (exogenous hormones), then adjusts the metabolism as needed, much like a thermostat. As it pertains to the testicles, the hypothalamus releases gonadotropin-releasing hormone (GNRH), which binds in the pituitary and triggers the release of luteinizing hormone. LH then travels to the testicles, aiding sperm production and turning up testosterone production.

If this hypothalamus-pituitary-gonad communication link is compromised, it can dramatically impact testicular function and testosterone. Testosterone inhibits feedback at the hypothalamus and can also be converted to estrogen via the enzyme aromatase. That estrogen plays a role in feedback to the pituitary, which is why the drug tamoxifen is sometimes used in men. The estrogen effect may come to be a major player here. We don't yet have proof, but many natural medicine practitioners, like myself, believe the sharp rise of low testosterone in young men may be connected with the estrogen saturation in our environment.

The hypothalamus and pituitary are also responsible for thyroid and adrenal function, which are all critical to metabolic function. We call them the HP-Axis: hypothalamus-pituitary-thyroid axis (HPT), hypothalamus-pituitary-adrenal axis (HPA), and hypothalamus-pituitary-gonadal axis (HPG, i.e., testicles and ovaries).

This is why some therapies, like HCG, can be effective in multiple ways for men. It's also why low libido and low testosterone issues, coming from the brain, usually result in fatigue, sleep disruption, mood issues, weight gain, cold intolerance, and more. When the hypothalamus "takes a hit," it negatively impacts multiple downstream processes in the thyroid, adrenals, and gonads.

Biochemistry

Remember, the nerve signals transfer into biochemical signals, including signaling molecules cGMP and nitric oxide. This is probably how testosterone gets involved in the regulation of erections. When the brain sends nerve signals to the penis, nitric oxide is released and signals cGMP. This then dilates blood vessels and sets the erection cascade in motion with increased blood flow in and decreased blood flow out.

cGMP is broken down by an enzyme called phosphodiesterase 5 (PDE5). Since PDE5 degrades cGMP activity, if it's overactive, blood flow into the penis is slowed and erection is either absent or incomplete.

This is how Viagra, Cialis, Levitra, and other erectile dysfunction drugs work. They each act as inhibitors to PDE5, prolonging action of cGMP activity, therefore allowing harder, longer-lasting erections.

This may also be where low testosterone comes in. Testosterone treatment increases nitric oxide activity and may stimulate the healthy promotion of erectile tissue.

Testosterone also may play a role in PDE5 inhibition because adequate testosterone levels are required for these drugs to work.

Testosterone is also having an impact on the brain. It's not completely understood how testosterone promotes libido and sexual function, but one of the hallmarks of any hormone is its ability to impact many enzymes and other hormone receptors involved in multiple areas. Testosterone is likely acting as a priming apparatus for the male sexual brain and penile function. Without this primer, the entire cascade is disrupted.

Blood Flow

Erectile dysfunction really boils down to a blood flow problem. When blood flow is compromised, erections won't happen. Blood vessel issues are particularly problematic for older, overweight men and those with metabolic syndrome or diabetes.

High blood sugar, high blood pressure, and inflammatory mechanisms are highly damaging to the cells lining the blood vessels. These are the same cells that are functioning through nitric oxide and cGMP. But the solution isn't to simply jump to testosterone and erection drugs. Taking testosterone in the context of an unhealthy lifestyle won't do a thing for you. Studies actually show complete restoration of erections in men as old as eighty when lifestyle is corrected.

Erection issues can also be early warning signs of cardiovascular disease. Fixing the issue at this stage requires a complete overhaul of diet and lifestyle. We're talking weight loss, decreased sugar and carb intake, weight training, and stress reduction. Continuing to live the couch potato life isn't going to get the job done.

THE TESTOSTERONE-SUPPORTIVE LIFESTYLE

For most healthy men under the age of fifty, the issue is likely going to be brain- or biochemistry related and not blood flow related. One of the first things you'll see with low testosterone is a lack of morning wood.

Again, most men will want to jump right to testosterone replacement therapy, but remember, hormones are like people and behave differently depending on the environment they're in. Make sure the overall biochemistry is the proper setup to have testosterone work correctly.

The first step is to live a testosterone-supportive lifestyle. The things that raise testosterone are:

- Adequate macronutrient intake. Get enough but not too much protein, fat, and carbohydrate.
- Adequate calorie intake. Not too much and not too little.
- Adequate intake of micronutrients. The three most important for testosterone may be zinc, magnesium, and vitamin D. Being low in any of these will compromise testosterone levels. Adding these in if you already have adequate amounts will likely do nothing, but correcting deficiencies will.
- Weight training and intense exercise. Lifting weights reliably stimulates testosterone. Intense exercise—high volume and heavy loads—is best.

- Enough but not too much exercise.
- Lots of walking, which sensitizes the body to insulin and lowers the stress hormone cortisol, both of which indirectly and negatively impact testosterone.

Insulin, Cortisol, and Testosterone

Because the hypothalamus is essentially a stress barometer, you don't want to train too hard, too often, or for too long. You also don't want to go to dietary extremes by cutting calories and/or carbs too low. Do enough but not too much—find that Goldilocks zone. Otherwise, you risk downstream negative effects flowing from a dysfunctional hypothalamus, which is negatively impacted by insulin resistance and excess cortisol.

Blood sugar management and insulin sensitivity are critical to testosterone. There's a hormone called SHBG (steroid hormone-binding globulin) that binds strongly to testosterone, effectively removing it from the usable pool of hormones.

Insulin resistance and excess cortisol both elevate SHBG. The end result is a reduction in usable testosterone, even when you're making enough. Not to mention, excess cortisol and insulin have many other negative effects that disrupt metabolic function.

Diet

Two dietary regimens useful for testosterone management are the 40-30-30 dietary strategy for heavy exercisers and athletes, and 30-40-30 for everyone else.

These formulas dictate the carb-protein-fat macronutrient ratios I typically use. If men are overweight, I suggest a calorie intake that can be calculated by multiplying your body weight times ten. For those training heavily, body weight multiplied times fifteen is a good starting point.

In other words:

- 10 × body weight and a 30-40-30 (carbs, protein, fat) diet for overweight, less active men
- 15 × body weight and 40-30-30 (carbs, protein, fat) ratio for all men engaged in frequent, intense exercise

I also suggest daily walks to sensitize insulin and lower cortisol, and weight lifting at least three times per week to promote testosterone. You can use this as a starting point, then ask yourself the following questions to see if you need to adjust anything:

- Is your HEC and other hormonal feedback (like libido and erection quality) improving?
- Is your body composition achieving the V-shape?
- Are your blood labs—free testosterone, total testosterone, and SHBG levels—improving?

If the answer to each is yes, you're on the right track. If not, start adjusting accordingly.

Testing and Labs

Once you get diet and exercise on the right track, a baseline of labs can help you see even more of the picture. I suggest getting:

- Testosterone, total and free
- SHBG

- Hemoglobin A1C (to rule out high blood sugar and diabetes)
- Fasting insulin (to rule out insulin resistance)
- DHEA sulfate
- Vitamin D
- High-sensitivity estrogen (to rule out high aromatase since some men aromatize testosterone to estrogen)

These should be done in addition to the general screening of lipids, CBC, and chem panel a doctor will do.

Some things you may want to consider:

- DHEA. Research has shown that 50 mg DHEA restores erectile function in 80 percent of males who are low.

- Vitamin D. Low vitamin D has been shown to impact testosterone, and restoring vitamin D to levels between 50 ng/ml and 100 ng/ml may raise testosterone to help with erections.

- Citrulline malate. This amino acid is a nitric oxide precursor. It can act as a weak Viagra, ensuring nitric oxide is abundant. An amount of 1.5 g per day improved erections in men within one month.

- Rhodiola. This one is controversial, but I've personally seen it to be effective. I've seen people reporting that rhodiola increased testosterone, libido, and erection quality. Given rhodiola's favorable effects on the hypothalamus, this makes sense. Take 200–400 mg a day. It may also help premature ejaculation. That makes sense given it's an adaptogen balancing the parasympathetic and sympathetic nervous system.

Hormonal Approaches to Raising Testosterone

Let's say you get your testosterone tested. What's considered low? Most standard reference ranges are:

- Total testosterone normal = 300–1,200 ng/dl. Many practitioners will treat if levels are below 500 and you have symptoms.
- Free testosterone = 5–21 ng/dl

A free testosterone below 10, and a total testosterone below 500 with testosterone-related symptoms, especially loss of morning erection, should be managed with the lifestyle changes and supplements listed above.

If there are no changes after three months of concerted effort, then, and only then, consider testosterone replacement therapy or TRT. Keep in mind, there's a difference between replacing testosterone and enhancing with testosterone. When you do TRT, you're seeking to restore normal levels, NOT trying to exceed them. Replacing to normal levels is not only beneficial for symptoms but likely one of the healthiest things you can do.

Enhancing with testosterone by going up 1,200 ng/dl isn't necessary and may cause some issues. Remember, what you want when restoring testosterone is to bring your levels back to optimal and help the hypothalamus-pituitary-gonadal axis become healthier. Raising testosterone to levels beyond physiological potential works against this goal.

If levels are low right out of the gate, you have two options: HCG monotherapy (and/or clomid) or testosterone replacement.

HCG Monotherapy

Human chorionic gonadotropin (HCG) is an LH analog, meaning it's biochemically similar enough to the LH hormone to interact with the same receptors. This means it can be used to turn on the testicular machinery, sperm, and testosterone production.

There are stories about HCG increasing ejaculation volume and increasing penis size. This can be true, but it may only be the case for those with hypogonadism or "micro-penis." The internet chat boards certainly aren't without their stories of slight enlargement with HCG in normal men. In the two studies I found on micro-penis, gains were three-fourths of an inch in length and girth.

HCG is a great option because, unlike testosterone, it may actually help the hypothalamus-gonadal axis as opposed to suppressing it. It also seems to have less impact on estrogen, prostate mass, and cardiovascular parameters compared to the more traditional TRT while being equal or better than TRT in raising testosterone.

This assessment is evidence based and taken from a well-done study on men aged forty-five to fifty-three with low T. The study compared HCG against transdermal testosterone and two different injectables.

Many doctors give HCG along with their testosterone therapies to keep the hypothalamus working and the testicles from shrinking. Why would the testicles shrink? Testosterone from an outside source turns off the hypothalamus's secretion of LH, and therefore the testicles stop producing sperm and testosterone. This is why ejaculate volume and testicles can shrink in men taking testosterone. This usually isn't a huge issue if the drug isn't abused, but HCG helps keep this from happening.

As an aside, steroids do not shrink the size of the glans penis (i.e., the shaft), just the testicles, and only if used in very high amounts for too long.

Using HCG alone is a reliable promoter of testosterone and may be the safer, more natural option to start with in those with HPG issues. It may also be the best approach for those who've been on testosterone for a long period of time.

Based on the studies, there are a few approaches here.

If using TRT, then the approach recommended is 250 IU of HCG taken as an intramuscular injection (IM) daily. If you're using HCG alone, according to the study above where it was directly compared to TRT, the dose is 2,000 IU per week.

Most doctors don't like giving such a high dose of HCG all at once for fear of excess estrogen production and desensitization of LH receptors. Although this study didn't show that, it may be a consideration.

Keeping a once-daily dose to 500 IU or less seems wise, which means you'd be injecting 500 IU one to four times per week (500 IU–2,000 IU) for HCG monotherapy.

Clomid

Clomid is another option. Clomid works by blocking estrogen hormone feedback at the hypothalamus. This increases natural LH production, which then stimulates testosterone production.

The dose for Clomid, at 25 mg per day or 50 mg every other day, has been shown to be effective in restoration of the HPG axis and very safe as well. At least in one study, Clomid compared directly to TRT outperformed testosterone treatment with no side effects of long-term use (up to forty months).

For those with secondary testosterone deficiency coming from the hypothalamus-pituitary axis, which is usually the case for younger men, HCG and clomid may be superior to TRT. Plus, the cost of clomid is vastly cheaper compared to TRT.

Testosterone Replacement Therapy

It's important to remember that steroids do not equal testosterone. Many people assume if they're taking anabolic steroids, they're taking testosterone. This is not the case.

Anabolic steroids can be testosterone or androgen derivatives. Drugs like Anavar, Trenbolone, Winstrol, Primobolan, and so forth, have anabolic and androgenic effects similar to testosterone, but they are not testosterone. This means they are not suitable for TRT. Such drugs are also frequently the culprit for erection issues and low testosterone, especially after stopping them.

These "non-testosterone steroids" will shut down the body's own production of testosterone, like any other steroid, but won't be able to replace testosterone's full effects in the body. These are best left to bodybuilding circles.

Another consideration is the creams, gels, and orals of the pharmaceutical world. You can't patent testosterone, so to make money off the therapy, drug companies tinker around with different delivery systems. These approaches are far inferior to injectable testosterone—I wouldn't use them unless you're completely averse to injections.

The main drugs to consider:

- Testosterone Cypionate
- Testosterone Enanthate
- Testosterone Propionate

There are two others: testosterone suspension and Sustanon. Testosterone suspension is 100 percent testosterone, while the three above are testosterone bound to esters that increase the half-life of the drug and make for slower absorption.

Suspension is rarely used due to the need for daily dosing and the rapid spikes and falls that occur with its use. Sustanon, too, is rarely used in medical circles, mostly because it's not as widely available. It's a mix of the different testosterones and is a great option if you can find it.

The different compounds bound to testosterone determine its half-life and therefore the dosing frequency. Cypionate is usually dosed one or two times per week (50–100 mg) as is enanthate (50–100 mg one or two times per week). Propionate dosage is every other day at 25–100 mg per day.

Everyone has their favorites. I prefer propionate > enanthate > cypionate. Propionate causes me to hold less water and just gives me a cleaner look and more even effects. You'll have to determine what works best for you.

Estrogen, DHT, and Hair Loss

The biochemical pathways involved with testosterone therapy also should be considered. Testosterone can be converted to estrogen via the enzyme aromatase. The use of aromatase inhibitors is beneficial in this regard, which is why many people will use Arimidex (anastrozole) along with their TRT.

Testosterone can also be converted into DHT, which may contribute to some side effects, including hair loss and acne. However, DHT may be a major libido enhancer. This occurs via the enzyme 5-alpha reductase, which is why Finasteride is often used with TRT as well.

The herbal world is filled with great aromatase and 5-alpha reductase inhibitors, often having both actions in one herb. I've found the use of products containing nettles, saw palmetto, pygeum chrysin, and DIM a reliable way to control these two biochemical pathways without pharmaceuticals.

Testing and Health

With TRT, we want to make sure we're not elevating prostate cancer and cardiovascular disease risks or other complications. You may want to consider monitoring prostate-specific antigen (PSA). This test is controversial but may be the best we have to assess prostate changes over time.

You'll also want to make sure hemoglobin and hematocrit levels aren't going up while on therapy. This can increase the risk for blood clots.

Finally, watch estrogen levels and the liver enzymes ALT and AST to make sure you're not over-aromatizing and the liver is handling the therapy, respectively.

Always take a close look at the free (direct) and total testosterone levels. If you're doing things correctly, you should see favorable changes in your blood labs on TRT. Cholesterol, triglycerides, blood sugar, and inflammatory markers usually fall.

Obviously, testosterone is a requirement for male health, and proper TRT should be improving energy, mood, libido, erections, and body composition while also making you healthier.

HORMONES AND SLEEP

For both men and women, sleep is the ultimate hormonal reset button. We all have a circadian rhythm regulating our sleep-wake cycle, and one of the best things you can do for your hormonal system is go to sleep and wake up at the same times each and every day. When you are constantly sleeping at odd times, you end up subjecting your body to light exposure when it's not supposed to have it, thereby wreaking havoc with your circadian rhythm and creating chronic stress.

We also have an ultradian rhythm, which causes our energy to peak in the morning and taper off beginning around noon. But there is an easy and effective way to give yourself an extra boost so you can remain active and productive throughout the rest of the day—naps.

Naps are best taken in the early afternoon between 1:00 p.m. and 3:00 p.m. They can be as short as a few minutes or as long as two hours—any more than that and you start messing with your sleep patterns. Research has shown that just a ten-minute nap can reverse many of the negative effects of a sleepless night. If you have more time, I recommend opting for ninety minutes, which will take you through one deep sleep cycle.

Although sleep plays a critical role in hormone balance and by default in metabolism, your stress level is perhaps the biggest influence on metabolism. One of the best ways to stimulate a healthy metabolism is to get your stress under control through movement and mindfulness. More on that later.

UNDERSTANDING HORMONE
AND METABOLIC "TYPES"

In reality, there are no such thing as "hormone types" or "metabolic types," at least not as far as science is concerned. The best way to think of these "hormone types" or "metabolic types" is as hormonal stages or metabolic states or even diagnoses. After all, what is a diagnosis if not assigning someone a "type" based on clinical symptoms and measurable laboratory disturbances? (More on diagnosis later.)

Take blood sugar, for example. We have those with normal blood sugar levels and normal blood sugar responses. We then have those who sometimes see blood sugar drop and suffer predictable signs and symptoms of hypoglycemia (fatigue, difficulty thinking, agitation, increased hunger, etc.). We call these people hypoglycemics. That's their type or "diagnosis." We then have others who have mild blood sugar impairments along with high blood pressure, elevated insulin levels, high triglycerides, and fat gain centered around the middle. We call this the metabolic syndrome type or prediabetics. Then, of course, we have diabetics type 1 and type 2.

The same could be said for thyroid. There are people with high thyroid function who suffer from anxiety, sweating, and increased heart rate and are usually thin with pronounced eyes. We call these hyperthyroid. Others have normal thyroid. They are called euthyroid. Then we have low-thyroid types. They are called hypothyroid. Sometimes we divide these into different types as well, based on the etiology. For example, we have primary hypo-thyroid, secondary hypothyroid, and Hashimoto's thyroiditis. These clinical entities are a form of typing. They are important for clinicians to understand so they can identify, stratify, and codify individual diseases. This allows the clinical entity to be studied and appropriate treatments to be determined.

As it pertains to women, think of it like this: clinically, we know that a normal menstruating woman has a particular hor-monal reality characterized by fluctuating estrogen and proges-terone. A pregnant woman is more progesterone dominant. A perimenopausal woman is more progesterone deficient with unpredictable estrogen (sometimes low and sometimes high). Clinically, these hormonal realities can help tailor lifestyle inter-ventions. Estrogen and progesterone influence hunger, cravings, energy, and more. Accounting for them aids the ability to sustain low-calorie diets and healthy lifestyle changes.

Women have two dominant sex steroids; men have one. Men go through only two hormonal stages (puberty and andropause); women can go through five (puberty, pregnancy, perimenopause, menopause, postmenopause). Men have more static levels of tes-tosterone throughout the month; women's hormones ebb and flow. All of this matters.

We know young women go through an estrogen-dominant phase and a progesterone-dominant phase each menstrual cycle. Perimenopause is characterized by lowering progesterone and fluctuating estrogen, menopause by low estrogen and proges-terone, and postmenopause by low estrogen, progesterone, and testosterone with relative testosterone dominance. Are these not useful hormonal realities?

Sex steroids impact other metabolic hormones (cortisol, insulin, thyroid, etc.) and influence hunger and cravings (due to effects on brain chemistry; estrogen impacts dopamine and serotonin while progesterone influences GABA). Taking these hormonal realities into account allows us to mitigate many of the compliance issues that plague most diet and exercise programs.

"Hormone types" are simply a best guess as to what lifestyle elements may be best to start with. They stratify women into buckets based on their life stage and hormonal symptoms. They are a form of temporary diagnosis. From there, the real work begins.

There are not seven different hormone types in women; there are infinite types. Each woman is unique in her physiology, psychology, personal preferences, and practical circumstances. By separating women according to their hormonal life stages, we provide some structure to begin. From there, we start the process of creating the lifestyle perfectly suited to their individual metabolic realities.

So there is no such thing as a hormone type, but you should probably still know yours.

CONTROVERSIES IN MEDICINE AND WITH METABOLIC TYPES

Let's speak a bit more on the concept of diagnosis. A diagnosis occurs when your physician does a physical exam, considers your symptoms, and evaluates your vitals and blood labs. Based on all of this information, they then attempt to pick out patterns and give your situation a name or label. This is important because medicine has characterized many types of diseases. Matching your symptoms, blood work, and vitals to a particular disease name allows doctors to treat you more effectively. That's because if your condition looks exactly like other people with the same condition, there is a body of research and case studies that might be helpful. Based on that body of research, there may be drugs that have been studied—depending on the diagnosis, there may even be a cure. Giving a diagnosis—or getting one—is one of the most important steps in treatment of a condition.

There is only one problem: most complaints don't have a diagnosis. Most things people complain of fall outside of the criteria required to properly name and codify what is going on. This is why eight out of the ten times you go see a physician for something like unexplained weight gain, fatigue, mood issues, or other generalized complaints, they will tell you, "There is nothing wrong" or "Everything is normal." At that point, your only option is to wait until things get so bad that a disease that can be named is discovered.

This points out one of the biggest flaws in conventional medicine. What can your doctor do for you if they can't diagnose you? The answer? Not much. And yet, we all know that long before a disease can be detected, there is dysfunction occurring. An example would be type 2 diabetes. In order for your physician to diagnose type 2 diabetes, they would need to see a fasted blood sugar value of 126 on two or more occasions. However, long before you reach those blood sugar values, the blood sugar numbers would have been creeping higher and higher all along. Maybe you had some symptoms, or maybe you didn't. Either way, at 126, you're diabetic, but at 120, you're not. Seems kind of silly, right?

That's where functional medicine comes in. Functional medicine is the specialty of doctors like me. We specialize in keeping people well, not just in treating the sick. We pay close attention to the subtle dysfunctions that occur far in advance of actual disease. This is tricky since without a diagnosis, we can't give a validated name to what people are experiencing. As a result, we use nondiagnostic descriptive terms like adrenal fatigue, sleep disturbances, menstrual irregularities, metabolic damage, estrogen dominance, and other terms you won't find in any medical diagnostics manual.

A few months back, I had a run-in with a physician on the internet. This doctor took issue with the idea of hormone types and terms like "estrogen dominance." He was an MD (medical doctor). Well, actually a DO (doctor of osteopathy). I am an ND (naturopathic doctor). In case you are wondering, these are all different types of doctors who work with patients. You can include chiropractors (DC) and physical therapists (DPT) and clinical psychologists (PsyD and PhD) in this as well.

Basically, he was behaving like a cop telling other first responders that they're useless. The problem with that is, cops aren't trained to put out fires and you don't want them trying to save your life in the back of an ambulance. Imagine a police officer who has taken an oath to protect and serve the public and instead spends their time attacking firefighters and paramedics to show who the better first responders are. That's how many health and fitness professionals behave on the internet.

MDs and DOs deal with drugs and surgery. Some ply in lifestyle medicine, but this is not their training. It's like a cop who learns CPR and advanced first aid. That's handy, but it's no substitute for the training of a paramedic.

In my opinion, one of the best things that has happened in medicine, health, and fitness is the number of different specialty doctors that are now available. There are those who specialize in diagnosis, drugs, and surgery. Those who specialize in injury rehab and joint health. Those who specialize in lifestyle medicine, supplements, and optimizing function rather than treating disease. All of these professionals serve a role and, like the first responders, do better by their patients when they work together.

So why am I going through all of this? I wanted to set the stage correctly for the discussion of female metabolism. Clinically, I use "hormone types" as a first step in stratifying women. It's the beginning step in helping them find their own unique type. If you are a woman, or a man who loves women, you should know it was not until 2001 that policymakers and regulating bodies in research and medicine realized women were drastically underrepresented in studies. At that point, these organizations put recommendations together to try to close that gap. Up until that time, research on health and fitness was almost entirely extrapolated from college-aged males. Recent research suggests not much has changed. In 2021, women are still often treated as small versions of men.

There is technically no such thing as a specific "hormone type." Each woman is uniquely different and so represents her own individual type. And as you know by now, it takes time, attention, mastery, and practice to finally uncover the individual metabolic makeup. In the meantime, however, it is useful to have subsets of types that represent a better starting point than simply guessing (i.e., a functional diagnosis). This is especially true of women because they have fluctuating hormones monthly. The idea with the female hormone types is to provide a starting place that more closely resembles her current hormonal/meta-bolic reality. Obviously, a young menstruating woman requires different considerations than a perimenopausal mature female. Understanding these different hormonal states is imperative if you are going to be effective in controlling metabolic outcomes.

Most women notice the hormonal fluctuations that go along with menses and the changes that occur during a regular menstrual cycle, through pregnancy, and then through menopause, but not all are aware of the precise way that estrogen, progesterone, and other hormones ebb and flow, thereby influencing all of the other hormones in their bodies, particularly the fat-burning hormones. Most women, particularly those with stable and predictable men-strual cycles, can actually make these hormonal changes work to their advantage when it comes to fat burning. Even if a specific hor-mone type doesn't apply to you, I encourage you to read this whole chapter as your hormonal balance and hormone type are bound to change over time. Understanding the different types will arm you with the critical information you need as these changes occur. Let's take a closer look at what's happening at each stage.

Normal Menstrual Cycle—Estrogen and Progesterone Balanced

The menstrual cycle begins with the first day of menses or bleed-ing. About halfway through (day fourteen), ovulation occurs. The egg is then available for insemination for an additional fourteen days, and the cycle repeats. For the first fourteen days of your menstrual cycle, progesterone is relatively flat. In fact, young women have similar amounts of progesterone in their bodies as men do prior to ovulation. During this time, estrogen slowly rises and peaks right around ovulation.

At this point in your cycle, you have more estrogen in your body relative to progesterone. This is called the follicular phase of your cycle because this is when the follicle that hosts the egg begins to develop. Two other important hormones influence the development of the follicle: follicle-stimulating hormone (FSH) and luteinizing hormone (LH).

Toward the end of the follicular phase of the cycle (right around day fourteen), you experience a spike in LH. This causes the follicle to rupture and the egg to be released. During this same period, the uterine lining begins to thicken under the influence of estrogen.

MENSTRUAL CYCLE

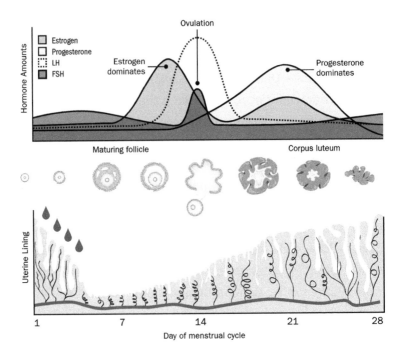

Once ovulation occurs and the egg is released, what's left of the follicle becomes the corpus luteum, which is the source of the name of the next part of the cycle: the luteal phase. The corpus luteum becomes the source of progesterone. So progesterone starts to rise and estrogen starts to fall after ovulation. Midway through the luteal phase, you end up with more progesterone than estrogen. There is still a lot of estrogen around, but it's not dominant as it was before.

If the egg is not fertilized and implanted (or attached to the wall of the uterus), progesterone and estrogen levels fall and the uterine lining is shed. Bleeding commences, and the cycle starts over.

As you can see, there is a natural ebb and flow of estrogen and progesterone throughout the cycle. The first fourteen days of your cycle is a time of more estrogen relative to progesterone. Then, after ovulation, there is a time of more progesterone than estrogen. Both hormones are still high, but progesterone dominates.

This ebb and flow of hormones, and the way it fluctuates throughout the life of a woman (from pregnancy through menopause), causes all the changes associated with female metabolism.

What this means is that if you learn to live, eat, and exercise in harmony with your hormones, you can take your fat-burning potential to a whole new level.

Normal Menstrual Cycle—Estrogen Dominant

Estrogen dominance occurs when you have too much estrogen relative to progesterone for too long. A younger woman who menstruates normally will be estrogen dominant in the first half of her cycle and progesterone dominant in the second half of her cycle. This is not a problem. In fact, this ebb and flow of hormones is exactly as nature intended.

However, if you remain estrogen dominant for too long, it can have many negative downstream consequences on your health, including fat gain.

There are really no good measurements for this that you can get at your doctor's office. Estrogen dominance is what we call a clinical manifestation—it makes sense, it is consistent with the science, but we don't have an accurate way of measuring it. However, we do know that estrogen dominance can occur for many reasons.

Estrogen Remains Dominant throughout Your Cycle

This can happen for many reasons, including not ovulating. Because the corpus luteum is the source of progesterone and it is only formed if ovulation occurs, lack of ovulation means no progesterone. The two major reasons this happens are stress and menopause. In fact, a young woman undergoing a lot of stress can push her metabolism into a state that closely resembles menopause.

It is useful to remind yourself that your female metabolism is exquisitely tuned to stress reactions. This is a requirement as your metabolism is built to prepare you for an optimal pregnancy. If it were not for the female metabolism's ability to finely tune itself to stressors, the human race would not have fared very well.

Too much stress, whether through chronic dieting, extreme exercise, or any other source, will register in your metabolism and disrupt the natural rhythm of estrogen and progesterone, leading to lack of ovulation and all the subsequent negative effects.

Chronic Stress

Chronic stress can place younger women in a menopause-like state also.

This happens for many complex biochemical reasons, but here is the short version. Chronic stress "agitates" the hypo-thalamus-pituitary-ovarian axis. This is the highway of information that runs from your brain to your reproductive organs and governs the whole process of menstruation and ovulation. When there is too much traffic on this highway or the traffic is "driving like crazy," it causes changes in FSH and LH and therefore can impact ovulation in ways that are similar to what we see in menopause. If a young woman is presenting with menopause-like symptoms, it's almost always a sign she is under extreme stress.

Environmental Toxins

We are awash in a sea of exogenous estrogens, meaning anything that comes from outside the human body. Exogenous estrogens are chemicals in the environment that mimic the actions of estrogen in the body. These endocrine-disrupting compounds are often referred to as persistent organic pollutants (POPs). They include things like pesticides, plasticizers, and industrial chemicals.

Some of these environmental hormones even come from our food and water. Milk is a major source of bovine (cow) estrogen and progesterone, and the global use of contraceptive pills may have made our water a source as well because when women ingest the pills, trace amounts of estrogen are urinated out. This is not completely removed by water treatment facilities, so it may end up in the water supply. The impact of this widespread estrogen in our environment is unknown, but it certainly can impact individuals who are most sensitive.

These estrogens have all kinds of consequences. Some can directly mimic estrogen, making your body think it has far too much of it. Others affect the estrogen receptors on your cells, blocking them so your real estrogen can't do its job.

When this happens, you can enter a state called estrogen resistance. Since some cells can't hear the message estrogen is trying to send and others hear the message too loudly, your body's own hormonal regulation gets confused and disrupted.

When your tissues can't hear the messages estrogen is trying to send, your body may begin to produce more and more of it. The usual outcome is that progesterone levels fall even further and take a back seat to estrogen effects. At this point, you enter a state of estrogen dominance, which can set off a cascade of hormonal imbalances.

As estrogen increases, progesterone may start to plummet further. Testosterone gets in on the action as well, often becoming relatively higher compared to progesterone and estrogen than it should be. This is when women start looking more like men, and you see patterns of male fat distribution (more fat around the belly) and hair growth (as can be the case with polycystic ovary syndrome [PCOS]).

The symptoms of estrogen dominance vary from woman to woman, but they include:

- Overproduction of uterine lining tissue
- Heavy periods
- Fibroids

- Endometriosis
- PCOS
- Pronounced hip, butt, and thigh tissue
- Being overly stressed out
- Anxiety and/or depression

Basically, what you end up with is a dysregulation of the hormonal symphony, with all kinds of bad downstream consequences. How do you get estrogen back into balance? Only by listening to your biofeedback and mastering your metabolism.

More on Estrogen Dominance

Under normal circumstances, estrogen is a powerhouse hormone in most every respect. It makes women more insulin sensitive. It makes women less cortisol reactive. It potentiates brain chemicals like dopamine and serotonin.

All of this means estrogen helps women feel more focused, driven, relaxed, and in control. It also means less hunger and better control over cravings. It means in a calorie deficit, women burn more fat and less muscle. And in calorie surplus, they gain less fat and more muscle.

Estrogen also is responsible for slower fat release around the breast, hips, butt, and thighs and faster release around the waist. This may sound less than ideal, but it's what gives women that beautiful hourglass shape.

So why are people always going on about too much estrogen? What exactly is estrogen dominance, and why is this term starting to show up in leading research articles in medical journals? Hormones work like a symphony. You don't want them too loud or too quiet. They must play at just the right volume, tone, and rhythm along with the other hormones. If they get too loud, off key, or out of sync, they can wreak havoc. When estrogen is in balance, everything is great. When it's out of balance, things start going sideways real quick.

In order for the female hormonal symphony to play in balanced harmony, there needs to be a natural hormonal ebb and flow between estrogen and progesterone. The first two weeks of the menstrual cycle, estrogen is off playing by herself, while her twin sister, progesterone, sleeps in late. Later, after ovulation, progesterone comes out to play with estrogen. Estrogen's influence is solitary the first two weeks, but in the next two weeks, progesterone and estrogen are high together with progesterone dominating.

If ovulation does not occur, which is common in stress and perimenopause, then estrogen levels remain dominant throughout the menstrual cycle. This is classic estrogen dominance.

There are other ways to become estrogen dominant. As we talked about above, organic pollutants often mimic estrogen in the body. These xenoestrogens act as metabolic disrupters. They mimic estrogen but not progesterone and cause excess estrogen effects. Again, this results in estrogen dominance.

A third way estrogen can dominate is via incomplete detoxification. When estrogen is taken out of circulation, it goes to the liver where it goes through a series of detox steps where it is put into the bile, secreted into the digestive tract, and hopefully pooped out. However, it can also get reabsorbed. If this happens, there are excess estrogen effects. Again, estrogen dominance.

In a final type of estrogen dominance, women may oversecrete testosterone. Testosterone acts much like a stress hormone in women, so this enhanced testosterone may occur with increased stress. It can also be genetic. Extra testosterone is often converted to estrogen in both men and women through a process called aromatization. And again, estrogen dominance.

So why is estrogen dominance an issue? When estrogen begins to dominate over progesterone, it goes from being a helpful metabolic hormone to a harmful one. Tissues that are estrogen responsive grow unabated. This leads to increased thickness of the uterine lining causing heavier, cramping, clotting bleeds. Like described above, it also can be the cause of fibroids, endometriosis, fibrocystic breasts, and ovarian cysts.

Estrogen increases thyroid-binding hormones and can induce hypothyroid symptoms as well. The balancing effect of estrogen becomes a disrupting factor if it is not in balance itself.

What can you do about estrogen dominance?

- Lower stress levels. Try to avoid being either overly fat or overly thin. ELEM (eating less and exercising more) and EMEL (eating more and exercising less) both cause stress to the system. Get adequate sleep. Don't overtrain. Take plenty of quality "me time." This will ensure that ovulation occurs and progesterone can balance out estrogen. Also consider female-specific adaptogens like Vitex to help the ovarian-brain connection work better.

- Eat more organic produce. This will elevate fiber and reduce intake of xenoestrogens. Fiber binds some of these estrogen-mimicking pollutants. And eating organic decreases exposure. Sweat therapy from sauna helps get rid of the pollutants already there.

- Eat even more fiber and perhaps take a supplement call calcium-D-glucarate. The fiber helps detoxed estrogen compounds bind and leave the body. Calcium-D-glucarate blocks an enzyme in the gut that reactivates estrogens.

- A healthy diet that adequately fuels exercise can help decrease stress and lower testosterone. There are also many natural products that are aromatase inhibitors including nettles, saw palmetto, chrysin, cruciferous veggies, and green tea. All can help lower testosterone-to-estrogen conversion.

Normal Menstrual Cycle—Progesterone Deficient

Whereas estrogen is a growth promoter, progesterone is a growth trimmer. If estrogen and progesterone were landscapers, estrogen would grow the hedges and weeds, and progesterone would trim the hedges and weed the garden. Estrogen and progesterone work together to keep the female physique lean and toned. Both hormones work together to keep fat from accumulating around the middle of the body. But when progesterone levels fall, this becomes much more difficult.

Progesterone interacts with receptors all over the body, including in the fat tissues, muscle cells, brain, ovaries, uterus, and breasts. So long as progesterone is in the Goldilocks zone, where everything is *just* right, everything works beautifully. But when progesterone drops too low, it can lead to issues.

When a hormone like progesterone declines, it impacts other hormones as well. For example, progesterone levels prime your tissues for other hormones to act—hormones like estrogen and thyroid. When progesterone levels decline, these other hormones are negatively impacted as well.

As a result, you may experience hypothyroid-like symptoms. These include cold intolerance, constipation, hair loss, decreased quality of skin and nails, thinning of the eyebrows, depression, fatigue, slow thinking, and memory issues. You may have periods of time when you feel tired, lethargic, and sluggish and other times when you feel wired, anxious, and buzzing inside.

Another area progesterone is crucial for is your brain and mood. Normal progesterone levels help maintain good levels of GABA, the number one relaxing brain chemical that calms you and helps you get to sleep. Low progesterone can cause GABA levels to fall, spiking anxiety and causing insomnia. The outcome of all of this is that you may be feeling confused and frustrated as to why things just seem slightly off. You may even experience ovarian cysts, irregular menses, and unpredictable menstrual symptoms and not have an explanation as to why.

You probably also notice a more difficult time keeping stomach fat at bay. Your body may feel flabbier and less toned. And the shape of your body may start to resemble something you no longer recognize.

Normal Menstrual Cycle—Estrogen and Progesterone Deficient

If you are estrogen and progesterone deficient, you have entered a state I refer to as ovarian burnout. Whether by choice or circumstance, your metabolic system is hyperactive and, as a result, has depleted the strength of both estrogen and progesterone. This often happens after a period of extreme stress, illness, dieting, or overexercising.

However, just as often, the stress is more silent and sneaks up on you without you realizing it. Typically when this happens, progesterone falls first, but if the stress continues, both hormones end up in a depressed flat line.

The female metabolism is very sensitive to stress. Too much stress to the female metabolism signals that it's not a good time to try to get pregnant. As a result, your metabolism becomes indifferent and uninterested. This is much like what ovarian burnout feels like as well—some days, you just want to lie in bed and do nothing or stare at the wall and veg. Being indifferent and having no energy feels like life just isn't as exciting or enjoyable as it once was. Believe it or not, lack of estrogen and progesterone can cause this.

It can also lead to fat gain and difficulty burning fat. Without progesterone's cortisol-blocking effects, you may see a redistribution of fat around your waist even if your weight does not change. This problem is compounded when you have a lack of estrogen because that hormone balances the effects of both cortisol and insulin.

Some women also experience hypothyroid-like symptoms when they are both estrogen and progesterone deficient. This is because both hormones influence the thyroid. As a result, you may be feeling tired but at the same time wired, with a lack of interest in things you used to love. You may feel you just don't have the energy or drive to do much at all. You may even lose interest in sex.

You will likely have short stints of feeling energetic, motivated, and focused, but more times than not, you will feel tired and wired with anxiety buzzing inside. But we can resolve those problems and rebalance your hormones, and this is precisely what you are learning to do in the pages of this book.

Perimenopause—Estrogen High or Fluctuating and Progesterone Deficient

When you move into perimenopause (the time just before you are in full-blown menopause), you will have times when ovulation does not occur. This happens, in part, because you get improper amounts of FSH and LH to help the follicle grow and mature. The outcome is that the follicle won't rupture. It also happens as the number of viable eggs becomes diminished. This means no egg (thus no ovulation), but it also means you don't get the corpus luteum.

Remember that the corpus luteum is the source of progesterone, so if it isn't there, your progesterone levels plummet. This can lead to extended periods of estrogen exposure without progesterone to balance it out. Sometimes estrogen will be dominant and take over the show.

At other times, it will become completely wiped out because it is never getting any help from progesterone. This is one of the reasons a person in perimenopause feels so unpredictable, uneasy, and unbalanced.

Under normal circumstances, estrogen and progesterone work together. Estrogen causes fat storage around the hips, butt, breasts, and thighs, and when acting with progesterone, keeps fat from being stored around the middle of the body. Both hormones also interact with receptors all over the body including in the fat tissues, muscle cells, brain, ovaries, uterus, and breasts.

When estrogen and progesterone are working together in harmony, they are responsible for helping create the often-desired hourglass body shape. But when progesterone is no longer exerting influence and estrogen is forced to do all the work itself, the latter's levels will rise and fall unpredictably.

When estrogen is high sometimes and low other times, the tissues it signals also become irregular in their function. One minute, the tissues and cells of the body see high estrogen, and the next, they see low, which can be rough on the metabolism.

Ultimately, perimenopause can feel incredibly random and can drive both your metabolism and mind crazy as you try to keep up. No two days will feel exactly the same. The chart on the following page shows just how wild the estrogen roller-coaster ride can be during perimenopause:

Your ovarian and uterine tissue are not getting the proper signals or rhythms anymore. Your periods will become irregular, unpredictable, lighter in flow, and fewer in frequency. You may notice your eating habits change as well. Although they may have been easier to maintain before, now it may be extremely difficult to manage unpredictable cravings and hunger that can range from ravenous to zero appetite at all.

You may also notice other areas of the body start to fare worse than before. Unpredictable digestion can ensue. Foods you tolerated previously may now cause heartburn or gas. You may find your thyroid and adrenal glands also take a beating. You may also begin to experience symptoms like bowel changes, cold intolerance, irritability, frustration, fatigue at some times and excess energy at others, all mainly due to the volatile nature of your fluctuating hormones.

CHANGES WITH PERIMENOPAUSE

The changes at perimenopause are almost exactly the same hormonally as when younger women are confronted with excess stress (yes, from extremes in diet and exercise too). Here are some things to consider and a few measures to take:

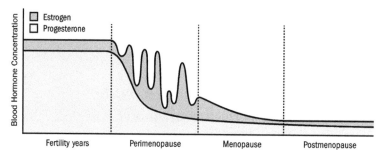

What Happens?

- As ovulation stops occurring, progesterone falls.

- Without progesterone signaling the hypothalamus and priming estrogen receptors, estrogen levels begin to fluctuate unpredictably.

- Estrogen and progesterone impact thyroid, cortisol, and insulin. So changes can occur in body fat distribution.

- Estrogen and progesterone impact serotonin, dopamine, and GABA. So brain chemistry changes can result in anxiety and/or depression, libido issues, hunger, cravings, and lack of motivation.

What To Do?

- Avoid extremes in diet and exercise.

- Use an intermittent diet approach rather than continuous or extreme calorie deprivation.

- Focus more on movement (i.e., relaxing walking) and less on intense exercise.

- Attend to stress reduction above all else!

One of the most impacted areas is the brain. Fluctuating estrogen levels create an unstable influence on serotonin and dopamine, leading to a lack of motivation and feelings of insecurity or depression. At the same time, low progesterone levels lead to falling levels of GABA. This, along with your estrogen levels bouncing around like a ping-pong ball, makes for an increased risk of worry and midnight monkey mind when you can't shut your brain off to go to sleep.

It is no wonder you are feeling so unstable, volatile, and out of balance—your hormonal system is partly to blame. But the good news is that by managing the 4Ms to accommodate for your fluctuating hormones, you can regain your energy, stabilize your mood, and even burn off the stubborn fat that piles up for many women during this period.

Menopause—Estrogen Deficient and Progesterone Deficient

As perimenopause progresses and you move into menopause, ovulation stops completely and estrogen starts to decline as well.

This means that both estrogen and progesterone fall over the course of perimenopause and menopause, but that doesn't happen on a nice smooth downward slope.

Instead, there are long periods of time when you have more estrogen than progesterone. This is very different than what happens during the normal menstrual cycle where there's an estrogen-dominant time and a progesterone-dominant time. This results in a period during which you're at risk for becoming more estrogen dominant because although both progesterone and estrogen are falling, progesterone is falling faster than estrogen, as the chart on the following page shows.

During this time, testosterone, insulin, and cortisol begin to have a greater impact because there is less progesterone and estrogen to buffer their effects.

During menopause, there's a decrease in estrogen, a decrease in progesterone, and an increase in testosterone relative to these two hormones, and you become more stress reactive and more insulin resistant. The result is a perfect fat-gain formula, and it's why many women pack on the pounds—especially around the belly—during menopause.

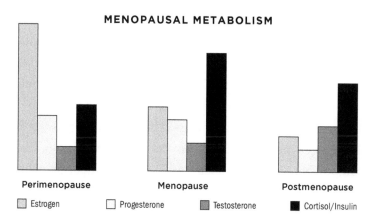

MENOPAUSAL METABOLISM

Perimenopause   Menopause   Postmenopause

☐ Estrogen   ☐ Progesterone   ▨ Testosterone   ■ Cortisol/Insulin

Menopause is three different states

Perimenopause: volatile estrogen (sometimes it's high and sometimes it's low) with falling progesterone

Menopause: estrogen falls along with progesterone leading to increased insulin resistance and increased stress reactivity (i.e., cortisol)

Postmenopause: estrogen, progesterone, and testosterone are low, but testosterone may be higher, relatively speaking

To add insult to injury, your brain chemistry changes during this time as well. GABA, your major relaxing neurotransmitter; dopamine, the brain-focusing chemical; and serotonin, your self-esteem and relaxing neurotransmitter, all decrease. One of the reasons this happens is because there are receptors for both estrogen and progesterone all over the body, including in your brain. Fluctuations in estrogen and progesterone levels therefore impact brain chemistry, and this can lead to mood changes and cravings, making it even more difficult for women at menopause to maintain their weight.

Postmenopause—Estrogen Deficient and Progesterone Deficient

After menopause is over and your cycle stops completely, you enter postmenopause. At this point, a woman's metabolism looks more like a man's with higher testosterone relative to estrogen and progesterone. There are two likely outcomes at this point.

If you weren't able to manage your weight during menopause, you will end up with extra fat—especially around the middle—and you'll have a harder time losing it because you are no longer in a position to take advantage of your unique female fat loss physiology. The other scenario is that you start looking like a man: you become more flat-chested and lose that hourglass shape.

The good news is that both of these situations can be managed by mastering your metabolism. If you learn to live, eat, and exercise in harmony with the hormonal changes you experience during and after menopause, you can not only maintain your weight but even burn fat.

SPECIAL CASES

Throughout life, many women will also experience several other different scenarios that can impact their hormonal balance. Pregnancy is a unique time in a woman's life when her metabolism acts slightly differently than it otherwise would. Some women never have normal cycles or suffer from other kinds of metabolic challenges. Let's take a look at some of these special cases.

Pregnancy and Metabolism

Most women view pregnancy as a time where their metabolism abandons them in favor of their growing little one. They almost resign themselves to a ruined metabolism postpartum and start strategizing how to deal with this reality after they give birth. But the truth is, pregnancy is one of the best things that can happen to a woman's metabolism—that is, if you do it right.

If the egg is fertilized and implantation occurs, HCG levels will rise and keep the corpus luteum around long enough for the placenta to take over progesterone production. Interestingly, HCG is the first hormone of pregnancy and is used clinically to diagnose pregnancy. After about eight weeks, the corpus luteum degrades and HCG levels fall off as the placenta takes on full-time duties of keeping estrogen and progesterone around.

Pregnancy is also a unique time as it is one of the few times in a woman's life when she remains progesterone dominant. The only other times are during the second half of the menstrual cycle and when a woman is breastfeeding. From pregnancy through breast-feeding is certainly the most extended period of progesterone dominance a woman experiences.

This has many implications, one of which is to increase glucose intolerance and promote insulin resistance. Remember, estrogen makes women more insulin sensitive, so when it is suppressed for any length of time, insulin resistance can result. This sounds bad, but remember that an insulin-resistant and glucose-intolerant metabolism means more food for the growing baby.

Of course, many doctors and health coaches completely get this wrong. The old advice of telling women to "eat for two" is not very sound. Your body is intelligent and will increase your hunger as needed without your conscious effort. By consciously going into pregnancy thinking you now have a license to eat as much and what-ever you want, you turn a great metabolic opportunity into a disaster.

It is estimated that a growing baby requires only about an extra 300 calories during the second trimester to 500 calories during the third trimester per day. There is no extra caloric requirement for the first trimester. There is no real need to count these calories, as your body will naturally and gently increase its SHMEC signals, allowing you to adjust your intake without much thought.

Studies show that more than half of pregnant moms gain more weight than is required for their pregnancy and subject themselves to metabolic issues like gestational diabetes along the way. Most expert resources give the following guidelines related to pregnancy weight gain:

- Underweight pre-pregnancy—BMI of less than 18.5 should gain 28 to 40 pounds

- Normal weight pre-pregnancy—BMI of 18.5 to 24.9 should gain 25 to 35 pounds

- Overweight pre-pregnancy—BMI of more than 25 should gain 15 to 25 pounds

The idea is to let the baby gain most of the weight while the mother adds enough fat and resources to sustain long-term breastfeeding. It is the combination of enough but not too much fat gain with breastfeeding that is such a powerful metabolic reset for women.

In fact, pregnancy can be a powerful metabolic reset. First, it allows the woman to relax and recover, provided they didn't have any significant or long-term complications. In fact, pregnancy is one of the only times relaxation and recovery are encouraged over the celebrated "stay busy and active" mindset of the Western world. Second, the progesterone dominance that persists through pregnancy and breastfeeding allows the body to be in more of an ELEL state without accumulating body fat because the extra calories are being used for the baby.

Breastfeeding

Assuming you follow a reasonable diet and exercise plan, you will supply your baby with all it requires, and you will set the stage for a metabolic reset once the baby is born.

It is important to understand two points here. First, this metabolic reset is contingent on breastfeeding for at least six months, but longer is probably better—nine to twenty-four months may be optimal. Next, breastfeeding will slow fat loss in the short term but significantly accelerate fat loss later.

Women who choose to bottle feed often end up losing weight a little faster than their breastfeeding counterparts, but after about three months, they are quickly surpassed by the breastfeeding moms. Breastfeeders are also shown to have leaner bodies—especially bellies and thighs—at all points after about six months. And those changes last.

One of the reasons for this has to do with changes your body goes through when you first start breastfeeding. Lactation requires your caloric intake to remain a little higher than it would be if you weren't breastfeeding. Again, there is no reason to count calories—your SHMEC will naturally dictate this.

During this time, the insulin resistance and glucose intolerance experienced during pregnancy reduce, but prolactin levels rise, and this hormone can slow fat release down a bit while lactating. All of this is beneficial and healing to the metabolism if you give it time and patience, and you eat, exercise, and live in a way that makes sense for what your body and your hormones are going through.

METABOLISM ISSUES IN FEMALES

What if you are one of the many women who do not follow the normal arc of menstruation, pregnancy, and menopause? What if you don't menstruate normally and haven't in some time?

Perhaps you have polycystic ovarian syndrome (PCOS), where your metabolism responds with a heightened stress response leading to insulin resistance, estrogen dominance, testosterone excess, and fertility issues. Maybe you suffer from the athlete triad—a state where the stress from exercise shuts down your production of estrogen and progesterone. Or you might suffer from some other condition that impacts your cycle.

In my experience, the keys to addressing such issues are the hypothalamus and the pituitary gland—the areas in the brain that are the command-and-control center for your metabolism. Your hypothalamus reads all the signals inside your body (from your thyroid, adrenals, ovaries, and more) and outside your body (temperature, exercise, emotional stress, diet quality and quantity), integrates this information, and sends messages to your body on the proper way to respond. This hypothalamus connection to the rest of the metabolism is known as the hypothalamus-pituitary axis or the HPA. It is sort of like the information highway for your entire body.

There are three major parts to it: the HPT (hypothalamus-pituitary-thyroid axis), the HPA (hypothalamus-pituitary-adrenal axis), and the HPG (hypothalamus-pituitary-gonadal axis—this includes the ovaries and testes). The HPA system is like a highly sensitive thermostat. When the body encounters metabolic extremes through illness, injury, or stress, this system reacts, creating metabolic dysfunction and damage.

Most of the women I have seen who are metabolically challenged suffer from imbalances in the HPA, whether it is due to PCOS, the athlete triad, or some other condition. Typically, when you focus on rebalancing the HPA, the problem disappears.

What Is PMS?

Premenstrual syndrome is believed to occur due to falling levels of estrogen and/or progesterone in the week leading up to menses. It is important to remember that there are receptors for estrogen and progesterone all over the body, including the brain, breast, muscle, and fat cells.

One theory about what causes PMS in some relates to the levels of estrogen that are always a bit more prevalent than progesterone. Remember that female metabolism is exquisitely balanced in its cyclical fluctuations of estrogen and progesterone.

Any change in this system—usually due to poorly designed diets or poor stress management—can result in symptoms of poor metabolic function.

As a result, SHMEC can go out of check and other uncomfortable symptoms can manifest including anxiety, depression, breast tenderness, cramping, and other effects. If you are a woman who has dealt with PMS, realize that this is an indication that your hormonal system may be out of balance, and you will want to use these symptoms as clues about how to design your new lifestyle. As you make progress, you may be surprised to see that these symptoms begin to dramatically improve.

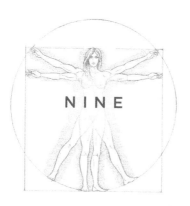

NINE

THE METABOLIC MASTER

B y now, you've learned how to master your metabolism by listening to the unique language it's always speaking to you through biofeedback. Although your body is capable of telling you part of the story, the rest becomes clear when you begin paying attention to what's happening in your brain. The way you treat your mind is just as important as how you treat your body when it comes to metabolism.

Consider metabolism's role as a stress barometer and how that has evolved over the span of mankind's existence. In man's early days, long periods of movement were nearly always followed by long periods of rest. That could mean regularly sleeping up to fourteen hours a day during the winter depending on the part of the world where one lived. Yet, even though the environment back then was not *go, go, go, go*, it was stressful in other ways. There was always the possibility they might not get food—or worse, they might become food. Moments of acute stress—sprinting after a wild caribou during the hunt or felling trees to build a temporary shelter—punctuated the daily routine of regular, slower movement and restorative downtime when they would walk for hours, then stop to sit under a tree or on a mountaintop. These intermittent moments of intense exercise forced humans to adapt and grow stronger.

The unpredictability of the environment forced our prehistoric ancestors to go without food for intermittent periods, which made rest something they simply couldn't sacrifice. They needed to conserve as much energy as possible so they were capable of the physical demands of finding food. They only had to deal with periods of chronic stress if they went too long without food and began to experience starvation, which we know is also the biggest stress you can put on metabolism.

Even though the human race has existed for thousands and thousands of years, it's only been in the last hundred or so that food has become readily available to most of us. Metabolism, however, is designed to conserve enough energy to procure more food, create a reserve, stay alive, and in the best possible scenario, reproduce. Humans were essentially built for long periods of movement in that perpetual search for food. For the last century or more, our metabolism has been functioning for a reality that doesn't reflect how we truly live; we no longer live in an environment where we have to constantly move in order to find enough food to stay alive. Today, most people's lives are exactly the opposite: they are rarely moving, they are ignoring their rest or recovery needs, they are eating all the time, and they are *constantly* experiencing some form of mental, physical, or emotional stress.

THE SCIENCE OF STRESS

Not only can stress hormones impact how many calories you eat in a day, but they can also impact the quality of calories you choose to eat and even influence how and where those calories might get stored or burned from. But what is the explanation for this? And more importantly, what can you do about it?

Hormones are cellular messengers in the sense that they deliver information about what's happening outside the body to cells inside the body, and cortisol is the 911 hormone. It triggers the body's first responders. Cortisol plays both a protective role and an adaptation role by working against inflammation and also releasing the body's sugar and fat stores to meet the demands of stress. Anything that poses a potential threat to the body will result in cortisol being called in to help.

I also call cortisol the Jekyll and Hyde hormone. If you recall from the story, Dr. Jekyll was a kind, upstanding citizen but was bothered at times with dark thoughts. This concerned him, and he developed a serum to disconnect himself from his dark impulses.

His attempt worked only partly, splitting his psyche in two and creating his alter ego, the evil Mr. Hyde. Ultimately, the story is about the struggle between the good, balanced side and the bad, extreme side.

I see cortisol the same way. Cortisol is "evil" in that it stores fat and shrinks muscle. However, it's also required for optimal health and actually burns fat, under the right circumstances. There's no question it can become destructive in certain situations, like when it's chronically elevated or continuously suppressed. When cortisol is too high or too low, it turns into the evil Mr. Hyde. When it's balanced, it becomes the helpful Dr. Jekyll.

Hormones also behave differently depending on the environment they are in and the people with whom they're surrounded. High cortisol in a low-calorie state will produce a different outcome than high cortisol in a high-calorie state. You want cortisol high while you're exercising; you want it low when you're not.

During exercise, cortisol works with your other fat-burning hormones, the catecholamines (adrenaline and noradrenaline) and growth hormone, to increase fat release. High cortisol levels when you're not exercising? That's a different story. When cortisol is "socializing" with insulin instead, it has the opposite effect.

Understanding these hormonal interactions is important. Technically speaking, cortisol is both a fat-storing and fat-burning hormone. This is because it increases the activity of lipoprotein lipase (LPL), the body's major fat-storing enzyme. But it also increases the activity of hormone-sensitive lipase (HSL), the body's chief fat-releasing enzyme.

Growth hormone and catecholamines, which are higher during exercise and fasting periods, accentuate cortisol's fat-burning potential while suppressing its fat-storing potential.

In the fed state, when insulin is around in high amounts, HSL activity is turned way down while LPL activity is cranked up. In this way, insulin magnifies cortisol's fat-storing properties while blocking its fat-burning activity.

Cortisol and insulin also block the action of each other by decreasing the sensitivity of their respective receptors. This means that eating is not the only way to become insulin resistant; stress can do it, too. So cortisol is actually not a fat-storing belly-fat hormone, despite what you may have been told. Insulin and cortisol together, with a high-calorie diet, are the real cause of belly fat.

Cortisol also interacts with the body's main metabolic fat-burning engine, the thyroid gland. Cortisol and the catecholamines sensitize thyroid receptors. Low cortisol can also lead to low thyroid activity. High cortisol blocks the normal conversion of inactive thyroid (T4) into active thyroid (T3). Again, much like Goldilocks, you don't want cortisol too low or too high, but just right.

HUNGER, CRAVINGS, AND FAT

There are two things required for fat loss—a calorie deficit and hormonal balance—and cortisol impacts both. Cortisol impacts several hormones responsible for hunger and cravings including leptin, insulin, and neuropeptide Y (NPY).

The command-and-control center of your metabolism is an area of the brain called the hypothalamus. This is the center of your metabolic sensor/thermostat. This area needs to "hear" the signals being sent by peripheral hormones like leptin and insulin, both of which shut down hunger in normal circumstances. Chronically elevated cortisol levels cause irritation in the hypothalamus, leading to downregulation of hormone receptors and inducing hormone resistance.

Imagine walking into a room with a strong odor and covering your nose and mouth, only to realize later you can no longer smell the odor. This is what cortisol does to the brain. It muffles its satiety-sensing mechanism. This makes it far less likely you will feel satisfied from meals and far more likely you'll eat more at current and future meals.

Cortisol also has an effect on cravings. By mechanisms not fully understood, cortisol, along with other stress hormones (i.e., the catecholamines), increases the desire for more palatable, calorie-dense foods. It does this while simultaneously shutting off the goal-oriented centers of the brain and ramping up the reward centers of the brain. This is a bad combo if you want to stick to your diet. In other words, there's a reason we want a triple-decker burger when we're stressed rather than the chicken and broccoli already prepared in the refrigerator. Cortisol may be the culprit.

On the other hand, NPY is one hormone produced by stress that even the most advanced experts know little about.

NPY is involved with hunger in the brain. But cortisol doesn't just impact brain NPY—it also impacts body NPY. When you're under acute stress, you release catecholamines and cortisol. When you're under chronic stress, you release more NPY. When catecholamines and cortisol are "socializing," they help you burn fat. But NPY makes you gain fat, especially when it's hanging around with cortisol.

When NPY is released in large amounts, it causes immature fat cells to grow into mature fat cells. Chronically high cortisol makes the body more responsive to this fat-storing action of NPY. In other words, NPY increases fat cell growth, and cortisol makes it more efficient at doing it.

Basically, cortisol combined with catecholamines, like it is in short-term stress, helps us burn fat. Cortisol combined with NPY, as it is in chronic stress, equals increased fat storage, especially around the middle.

Cortisol is made in the adrenal glands mostly, but it also thrives in belly fat. The deep fat of the belly, called visceral belly fat, contains an enzyme called 11-beta hydroxysteroid dehydrogenase (11-HSD). This is an enzyme that converts inactive cortisone into active cortisol. In other words, belly fat can produce its own cortisol.

In yet another twist in the complicated relationship between insulin and cortisol, insulin increases 11-HSD activity, which increases cortisol levels, which then causes increased insulin resistance. In this way, belly fat acts like a parasite ensuring its growth at the detriment of the host. This is important because often, stubborn belly fat remains despite best efforts with diet and exercise. Sometimes an extra hour in bed, to lower cortisol, may be a better strategy than an extra hour on the treadmill.

Cortisol Management

The three best ways to control cortisol are diet, exercise, and lifestyle. And the easiest way to assess if cortisol is balanced is by paying attention to hunger, energy, and cravings (HEC). If HEC is in check, it's likely cortisol is as well. The following are a few ways to make sure that's the case.

Eating Frequency

Remember, cortisol is an alarm hormone, and both eating and not eating can raise cortisol levels. Skipping meals can raise cortisol because the brain requires a constant supply of glucose. For some, skipping meals will cause blood sugar changes that create a cortisol response, and doing this too much can start causing many negative effects. Eating also can raise cortisol. Again, cortisol is the alarm hormone and helps regulate the immune response. In those who have food sensitivities, this effect can be pronounced.

When it comes to eating frequency, it's important to let research refine your approach, not define it. Eat frequently enough to keep your HEC in check. For some, this may mean consuming lots of small frequent meals. For others, it may mean fewer, smaller meals.

There is no one size fits all here. Just remember that a healthy low-calorie meal is neither healthy nor low calorie if you find yourself crushing half a cheesecake at the end of the day. And although there's a lot of controversy over meal timing, one possible benefit to a postworkout recovery drink is the quick suppression of postworkout cortisol.

Exercise

Short, intense exercise, or exercise that's weight training dominant, and slow, relaxing exercises are best for cortisol. In the case of short, intense exercise, cortisol is elevated along with growth hormone and catecholamines, which is good for fat burning. Plus, the shorter duration may mean less compensatory hunger later and less chance of going catabolic.

With longer-duration moderate and intense exercise, cortisol can easily dominate over the growth-promoting hormones and be associated with more postworkout hunger and cravings and less anabolic potential. Is this the reason sprinters and marathoners look so different? Probably not entirely, but after accounting for genetics, it's not a huge jump to suggest this mechanism is playing a role.

Another great way to lower cortisol is finishing workouts with slow, relaxing movements like leisure walking, which is even more impactful when done in nature.

Rest-Based Living

Find as many opportunities as possible to prioritize R&R workouts. These include naps, sex/physical affection, massage, foam rolling, laughter, time with pets, leisure walking, sauna, hot baths, contrast showers, meditation, and so on. All of these activities have applications in lowering cortisol.

THERMAL CHALLENGES AND TOXIC EXPOSURES

Two of the most insidious stressors for modern man come from constant, nondeviating temperatures and environmental endocrine disruptors. For early man, living in natural conditions meant the metabolism was constantly confronted with the task of turning body temperature up or down. Cold exposure generated mitochondrial shifts to not just making energy but also generating heat (called mitochondrial uncoupling). This is very much like an inefficient car engine that overheats easily. When the body needs to heat itself up, it diverts some of its energy production resources to the generation of heat. That process uses significantly more energy than is expended in normal situations. Cold exposure turns on shivering and slowly alters the physiology of pockets of fat tissue to become more muscle-like (called brown fat or beige fat). This also has an energy cost associated with it. The same is true when exposed to heat; sweating is more costly energetically speaking than not sweating.

Research hints that these thermal challenges, when added up over the days and weeks, become a huge energy sink, making calorie deficits much easier to achieve through an uptick in resting energy expenditure and non-exercise-related activity. Modern man has completely circumvented this through constant heating and air keeping ambient temperatures at a comfortable room temperature (20°C, 72°F). This is one of the reasons I have used sweat therapies such as hot baths, showers, exercising in hot settings, and saunas (the last being the easiest and most efficient), along with cold exposures such as cold showers, cold plunges, cold walks with minimal clothes, and cold sleep, which entails turning the AC down at night or use of high-tech beds and bedding that cool the body down.

One confounding aspect of this important metabolic tool is the compensatory nature of the metabolism. As you now know, the metabolism is adaptive and reactive, not linear or static.

Science confirms that thermal exposures can have many positive benefits on metabolic health, but they do not always result in weight loss. Remember, thermal stress speeds up metabolism. That also speeds up hunger and cravings for most. For ancestral humans, this was not an issue as overconsuming food was not the problem. In fact, this increase in hunger and cravings was highly beneficial as a motivating factor to get them out from under the shade tree or the warm cave and back out into the elements. In other words, thermal stress was naturally coupled to hunger and movement in a way that is not true of modern man. It's important to keep this in mind when using these metabolic tools.

Hot and cold therapies have many other benefits in keeping the metabolism healthy and flexible, including priming of the hypothalamus-pituitary-adrenal/thyroid/gonadal axis. These hot and cold exposures act as a stimulus for adaptation through the production of heat and cold shock proteins, eliciting certain hormonal effects (insulin sensitivity, growth hormone, etc.) and most interestingly, genetic transcription factors that turn on metabolic repair and anti-aging genes. In fact, the alternating use of hot and cold therapy (i.e., hot sauna alternated with cold plunges or showers) acts like an adaptogen for the metabolism. Adaptogens are unique tools that increase low metabolic function and lower raised metabolic function. In other words, they help the metabolism stay in the coveted Goldilocks zone. I have used this therapy to restore metabolic function to many patients and would recommend anyone seeking to attain and maintain a lean, healthy, and fit metabolism invest in a sauna and some type of cold exposure apparatus.

Finally, hot thermal exposure makes you sweat. Our metabolisms have a huge number of chemical compounds in them, things like PCBs, phthalates, heavy metals, organochlorines, and more. These POPs (persistent organic pollutants) get sprayed on plants, released into air, or dispersed in water. Animals then eat the plants, breathe the air, and drink the water. We then eat the animals and plants and drink the water and breathe the air.

These compounds act as chemical disruptors in myriad ways, two of the most important being as leptin antagonists and thyroid disruptors. Leptin is a major metabolic control hormone. It turns up and down the metabolic rate through adrenal and thyroid hormones and turns up or down hunger in the brain. These chemicals disrupt this delicate signaling system. They also cause multiple disruptions in thyroid production, elimination, and action. None of this is good or healthy. This is another "hidden" metabolic disruptor, and sweat therapy is probably the best way to get rid of these compounds. When researchers analyze other routes of elimination such as feces, urine, and breath, they find the widest array and highest concentrations of these compounds are showing up in perspiration.

This is why thermal exposures, most especially sauna and sweating, are so critical to metabolic health and function. You can think of these as passive forms of adaptogenic stress. Short-term, acute stress is very different than chronic stress. Acute, short-lived stressors help the body adapt and get stronger, and the body becomes more resilient and flexible as a result. Chronic stress degrades the system, creating a rigid and stagnant metabolism that moves into protective mode.

MIND OVER MATTER

The human body is one big stress barometer. Your metabolism is designed to do one major thing: measure and react to stress. This is why your mindset around stress is so important, yet almost no one pays any attention to it.

How many times have you heard someone say, "You know, I'm having trouble losing weight. I should take a nap or a hot bath or go have some relaxing sex"? My guess is never. In fact, most people typically do the opposite. They say, "I need to take this supplement, drink this magic elixir, do the latest exercise craze twice daily, and eat nothing but organic kale and wild line-caught salmon." None of that is addressing the real underlying issue.

If stress is the problem, having a healthy mindset around a lifestyle of rest, recovery, and relaxation is the solution. Let's look a little closer at stress and how it can kill your results.

STRESS AND FAT GAIN

How many calories does stress have? That might seem like an odd question, but ask almost any health and fitness expert if stress can make a person fat and you will hear a resounding yes. But if we agree that stress has no calories and we also believe that fat gain is about nothing but calories, then how exactly does stress stimulate fat gain?

Stress and other lifestyle factors work through complicated hormonal and metabolic mechanisms that alter not only the number of calories we eat and where on the body we store them but, most importantly, which type we burn: sugar, fat, or muscle.

Since the beginning of our existence, humans have been designed for acute stress like running away from a hungry predator, fighting off an intruder, or catching dinner. Your physiology is hardwired to the realities of your historic ancestors. Whether you are being chased by a pack of wolves, fighting a wild boar, under a severe deadline at work, facing financial uncertainty, or stuck in traffic, your response to stress is exactly the same as far as your physiology is concerned.

The stress response is regulated by closely orchestrated communication between the hypothalamus, the pituitary gland, and your adrenal glands. Think of the brain as an army's central command center. When it gets a warning that there is an incoming threat, it sends an immediate signal to the adrenal glands. In a fraction of a second, the adrenal glands flood the body with hormonal signals like adrenaline, noradrenaline, and cortisol, whose job is to give the body the energy required to stay and fight or run like hell.

You know what this feels like. If you have ever been in or near a car accident, you probably felt an intense surge of energy travel through your body that allowed you to slam on the brakes or swerve out of the way. That was your HPA axis in action. This is where things can go wrong.

In the modern day, there is nothing to run from, no immediate threat, no giant beast you have to kill to get lunch. So instead of moving in response to stress, you just sit there with large amounts of adrenal hormones surging through your body, which is not good. The major action of adrenal hormones is to raise the amount of sugar and fat in the blood to supply the body with energy. The whole body mobilizes all at once to supply the body with everything it needs to survive. The liver is instructed to kick out stored sugar as well as make some extra. Muscle and fat aid the creation of new sugar through the release of amino acids from muscle and glycerol from triglyceride (fat), respectively.

In other words, stress burns fat, sugar, and muscle under normal circumstances. But when it becomes recurrent and chronic, fat is usually spared while muscle is taken. Historically, when your body became stressed out, you were able to run your way to safety or fight your way out of danger. The process of intense movement to run away or fight is just what the body needs, because that triggers the release of other hormones like testosterone and human growth hormone (HGH).

Those hormones act to repair damaged tissue and partition energy usage toward fat metabolism while at the same time sparing and even building muscle. The repair mechanisms of these two hormones rebuild the body leaner, faster, and stronger, improving the chances that the next stressful encounter will result in another success.

All of this together feeds back on the brain and the adrenals, allowing them to stop the alarms and go back to a rest and recovery physiology.

The problem starts when stress, whether real or perceived, becomes constant and continuous, is not followed by intense activity, is not controlled through relaxing walking, or never ends. Chronic stress is different because the stressors continually force the body to work harder and harder to compensate for the physiological disruptions.

One of the first and most important things to change is the relative amounts of cortisol in your blood. "Relative" is an important term because it means how much cortisol you have in relation to other hormones.

The most important thing to remember here is that cortisol exerts actions on the body beyond your awareness. High amounts of continuous cortisol secretion induce serious changes in your physiology. Two important changes occur in relation to hunger and cravings. Excess cortisol impacts hunger and increases the urge for sweets and fatty foods. A sure sign that you have high stress levels is a lack of appetite in the morning.

Cortisol can decrease hunger in the short term and increase binge eating with a desire for highly palatable foods later. In other words, cortisol makes you eat less often but makes you overeat the wrong foods when you get the chance. This makes complete sense when you think about stress from a historic perspective. If walking out of your house could result in you getting swept away by a giant pterodactyl, you would likely make fewer trips to the grocery store and seek out the most energy-dense foods to sustain you for longer. In other words, you would eat less frequently and avoid the danger lurking outside as much as possible.

A comprehensive review by Dr. Pecoraro of UCLA San Francisco was published in 2006 in the journal *Progress in Neurobiology*.[38] In that paper, he cited research that showed that this is exactly the case.

The review showed that through several overlapping mechanisms, chronic stress caused animals to decrease the number of times they ate, opting for a few big meals over lots of smaller ones. Stress also forced a preferential desire for sugar and fat over regular mixed-composition meals.

The study showed that this happens at the level of the brain, because glucocorticoids, like cortisol, affect brain chemicals, specifically dopamine and opioids. These can lead to depression or anxiety, lack of motivation, lack of spontaneous movement, and a desire for high-calorie foods. Sounds a lot like what we call emotional eating, right?

The bottom line here is that stress, when chronic and persistent, affects brain chemistry in a way that changes behavior. These behaviors are directly correlated to obesity and appear to be coming from more unconscious centers of the brain.

STRESS AND WOMEN

Stress is definitely a menace when it comes to metabolism, and it is even more an issue for women. You have to remember that your metabolism is a stress barometer, and as a woman, one of the major things it is measuring is the safety of diverting resources to reproduction.

If the metabolism deems things are "too stressful," it begins to downregulate the female hormones. Typically, progesterone drops first, which removes some of a woman's ability to cope with stress and begins to make estrogen less effective as well (progesterone primes estrogen receptors and vice versa).

Next, estrogen falls, leaving the female metabolism exposed to the full onslaught of cortisol and chronic stress as described above. This is one of the reasons why taking diet and exercise to the extreme is a huge contributing factor in the lack of results in body change and may be the major cause of fat gain or the inability to lose fat.

The most important thing a woman can do to control the situation is to listen closely to what her body is telling her at each stage of her life.

MENSTRUATION MINDSET MODIFICATIONS

The body handles stress in unique ways, and one of the ways it can impact some people is to make the metabolic seesaw shift in unexpected ways. This causes the command-and-control center of your metabolism—your hypothalamus—to send signals to the thyroid, adrenal glands, and ovaries.

This can compromise your hormones even further, and you can end up in a downward spiral of metabolic dysfunction.

As a younger woman with a normal cycle, your estrogen and progesterone levels are exquisitely attuned to this, and that can be a problem. We live in an environment that is stress-heavy, and most of us typically prioritize doing more and going harder over resting appropriately and working smarter.

I like to think of the ovarian system as a woman's most sensitive stress barometer. As stress levels rise, ovarian function becomes compromised. This results in falling progesterone, fluctuating estrogen, and then complete ovarian fatigue.

What you need to do is adjust your 4Ms so that you are reducing stress exposure, combatting stress excess (through relaxing and restorative behaviors), and not overdoing diet and exercise, which you may be prone to.

There are many things you can do to reduce stress: meditation, massage, naps, sleep, hot baths, sauna, tai chi, relaxing stretching, and a lot more. However, there are some specific activities that can benefit your stress levels depending on your hormone type.

Normal Menstrual Cycle—Estrogen and Progesterone Balanced

In your case, stress is not much of an issue in the first half of the month but begins to really make an impact in the weeks leading up to menses. To help balance that, we want to do things to decrease stress, especially in the premenstrual period.

Two things that might be especially useful for you are walking in nature and warm Epsom salt baths. Relaxed, slow-paced walking is able to lower stress, and doing this in green areas is even better. When you add Epsom salt to your bath, it takes an already wonderfully relaxing activity and puts its stress-reducing effects into overdrive. Epsom salt is magnesium sulfate, and magnesium is very relaxing to the nervous system. Both of these things dramatically counter stress and keep the hunger and cravings at bay.

In the two weeks leading up to menses, I encourage you to either take a thirty- to ninety-minute walk, preferably in a green setting, or take a long, relaxing bath. Do this every day, and you will be priming your metabolism to respond in a way you never imagined.

Normal Menstrual Cycle—Estrogen Dominant

There are many ways you can become estrogen dominant. Regardless of how it happens, decreasing stress will help you rebalance your estrogen levels.

Hot baths and/or sauna therapy may be particularly helpful if this is the case for you. These therapies get you sweating, which is one of the main ways you get rid of some of the persistent organic pollutants, or POPs, that can have estrogen-like effects in the body.

I suggest you begin taking a hot bath or sauna—hot enough to get you sweating but cool enough to remain relaxing and allow you to sweat lightly—for twenty to sixty minutes. Do this at least three times per week and preferably five or six times per week.

Normal Menstrual Cycle—Progesterone Deficient

In your case, this command-and-control signal may be getting jumbled a bit because progesterone levels are required to keep this entire system prime and sensitized. If progesterone levels fall, this system can become less dependable and more prone to issues.

In this case, it's important to decrease stress or at least lessen its effects. This is the best way to maintain adequate progesterone levels. A great way to start is by learning to use your breath to adjust your physiology as needed. You can calm your mind by focusing on your breathing. This can produce a relaxation response in your brain and body that will wipe the stress away.

I recommend the following technique:

- Take a deep breath.
- Count eight seconds on the inhale.
- Hold your breath for two seconds.
- Exhale for four seconds.
- After completing this for ten breaths, close your eyes, take a big deep breath in, and hold it for as long as you comfortably can.

Use this time to reset your senses and still your mind. Listen to your heartbeat or watch the color changes dance around in the back of your eyelids. Repeat this up to three times per day, including before bed to help you sleep.

Normal Menstrual Cycle—Estrogen and Progesterone Deficient

In your case, the command-and-control signal has either lost its ability to communicate to the ovaries, or the ovaries have lost their ability to respond. It is almost always a combination of both, but most issues start in the brain and end in the ovaries.

That is why we want to do things to decrease stress and reduce its effects on the brain first. This is the best way to reboot the ovarian system and get estrogen and progesterone back in line.

Getting your body in restorative relaxation mode is going to be the key. You can think of this as a reboot to your metabolic hard drive. The best way to do that is to sleep. There is only one problem—of all the hormonal types, you may have the most difficult time getting to sleep at night. To combat this, you can use two other reboot techniques alongside sleep: naps and meditation.

Just a ten- to thirty-minute nap can undo many of the hormonal problems caused by sleep loss. Meditation has also been shown to restore function in the body and brain similar to how a nap does. By focusing on your breath, I mean counting the breaths. In, then out—that's one. Continue focusing on and counting your breath until you reach a count of ten, then start back over at one.

If your mind wanders and you forget your count, just go back to one. The counting allows you to catch your mind when it drifts. Mental drift is normal in meditation, and with practice, you can focus for much longer.

I want you to prioritize sleep by taking three steps:

- First, go to bed one hour earlier and rise one hour later to start. Shoot for nine hours of sleep every night.
- Second, take a brief ten- to twenty-minute nap between the hours of noon and 4:00 p.m. five days a week.
- Finally, meditate for five minutes by focusing on your breath at least three times per week.

MENOPAUSE MINDSET MODIFICATIONS

Due to fluctuating estrogen and falling progesterone during this time of life, your entire system is forever losing its cyclical rhythm. This means that you are now becoming more sensitive to fat storage from food and more reactive to fat storage from stress. It's a double whammy.

Learning how to cope with stress more effectively is essential. That being said, the modern Western lifestyle has a completely dysfunctional attitude toward stress. It is crucial that you do things to reduce your stress load. You can try meditation, massage, naps, sleep, hot baths, sauna, tai chi, relaxing stretching, or anything else that helps you unwind and recenter.

Although all of these can help, I can offer specific suggestions based on your hormone type.

Perimenopause—Estrogen Fluctuating, Progesterone Deficient

One thing that might be especially useful for you is any social activity with friends that involves engaging in relaxing treatments like spa facials, pedicures, and massages. Social support is critical during this time of life as it helps buffer against some of the unpredictable symptoms you are dealing with.

Spending more time with friends going through the same thing is a great way to vent, connect, and reduce stress. Try doing this while getting your nails done, getting a massage, or doing anything you can do to treat yourself and relax. You'll get double the benefit. Plan at least two to four relaxing social outings with friends and/or family per week. Walking groups are great for this, as are creative groups like book clubs or other creative outlets.

In addition, I want you to engage in spa treatments as much as possible—at least three times per week. I realize this can become an issue in terms of time and finances, and I don't want you to stress about that. If finances are an issue, look for lower-cost alternatives such as self-massage and stretching classes like restorative yoga.

Menopause—Estrogen and Progesterone Deficient

As estrogen and progesterone levels drop, your already exquisitely attuned stress barometer gets even more sensitive because you become more reactive to the stress hormone cortisol. Reducing stress is the best way to deal with this new reality of reduced estrogen and progesterone. But our society doesn't make that easy.

Probably the most important thing a woman in your time of life can do to get her body in restorative relaxation mode is get enough sleep. Sleep is like a reboot to your metabolic hard drive. However, you may have great difficulty falling asleep at night due to your changing hormones. This is where naps and meditation again become especially important.

I again encourage you to try to go to bed one hour earlier and rise one hour later to start, aiming for nine hours of sleep every night, in addition to adding in ten- to twenty-minute naps between noon and 4:00 p.m. five days a week and meditating by focusing on your breath three times a week.

Postmenopause—Estrogen and Progesterone Deficient

At this point in your life, age has caused your ovaries to lose their ability to respond to the demands of your metabolism. That means that you need to learn how to anticipate those demands and take action to respond.

Here again, sleep is the number one best stress reducer you can engage in at this stage. And yet again, you may find it harder to sleep now than you did in your younger years due to the changes in your hormone levels. Just remember that when sleep is problematic, naps and meditation work wonders. Give yourself time and permission to take care of yourself by doing both.

REST-BASED RECOMMENDATIONS FOR ALL

Of course, your options for relaxation go way beyond those outlined for your specific hormone type. The solution to a stress-filled life lies in understanding that the fast-paced, get-it-done-now, never-take-a-break, harder-faster-longer mindset is the problem. Lifestyle choices matter. There are many choices you can make that lower stress hormones and help the metabolism get back into balance.

Connection Therapy

Laughing lowers cortisol. This is why time with friends, connection to family, hanging with pets, and anything else that puts you in a happy mood is key.

Sex and cuddling, both separately and more powerfully when combined, are powerful stress reducers.

Orgasm, whether through masturbation or sex, immediately puts the metabolism in relax and recovery mode. Add a long cuddle to that and you are in stress-relieving bliss.

Water Therapy

Long showers and relaxing baths are an excellent option.

Relaxing spa-like music with candlelight is a perfect way to amplify the stress-relieving benefits of water therapy.

Hot baths are a wonderful way to detoxify your body, eliminating toxins through sweat while relaxing. Sweating, in particular, may be especially beneficial to a subset of persistent organic pollutants or POPs. These compounds can act in the body as hormone disruptors and therefore their removal has the potential to rebalance hormone function.

Relaxation Therapy

Get plenty of sleep. Sleep deprivation elevates stress hormone production and sends SHMEC out of check.

Take naps. Just ten minutes can undo much of the dysfunction associated with sleep deprivation. And it is much better than adding in another workout.

Get a massage. Massage has benefits due to its ability to focus the mind on the present, relax the metabolism, and release muscular tension and strain. Even self-massage techniques like foam rolling are wonderful for stress.

Practice meditation. The relative contribution of sympathetic (stimulating) and parasympathetic (relaxing) activity is balanced out. Mindfulness has also been shown to help those who practice it become more stress resistant over time.

Movement Therapy

Avoid heavy exercise. Intense physical activity typically is not relaxing, so you don't need to do more than what is comfortable for you.

Relaxing and stretching yogas are great as is tai chi. Aim for activities that integrate mindfulness and slow rhythmic movements of the body. The outcome is very similar to walking in its ability to calm and center the metabolism.

Speaking of which, take a walk. Walking lowers cortisol so long as you are going at a leisurely pace, not huffing and puffing through a power walk. If you do it in nature, all the better.

The idea is to schedule these rest, recovery, and relaxation sessions into your daily life as much as possible. Specifically, making walking the central focus of your stress reduction and then using other modalities daily or even multiple times per day are going to make all the difference in the world.

Find and use as many different tools and techniques as you can. The modern day provides increasing options in this regard. Spas, deprivation chambers, massage therapists, saunas—the list goes on and on. The point is to find what works for you and do it. Use the techniques to decrease your stress output and your body will thank you.

MOVEMENT VERSUS EXERCISE

Movement is one of the only forms of activity that lowers stress hormones while sensitizing the body to insulin, and in general, it's incompatible with food—in other words, you're rarely eating while moving. Movement is also an independent means of getting fuel into the muscles without the need for insulin. Because movement calms and sensitizes metabolism, it is extremely useful for recovery, and rhythmic or meditative movement can elevate mindfulness.

It also is simply good for your overall health. Research has shown that inactivity may be the biggest risk factor of all for diabetes and heart disease, two of the end-stage consequences of a damaged metabolism. In one study published in the May 2013 issue of the journal *Diabetologia*, researchers showed that movement was a far better predictor of health than either moderate or even intense physical exercise.[39] In other words, sitting all day long and then going for a vigorous thirty-minute run was not nearly as effective for health and metabolic function as just moving more.

This research, and other studies like it, have led many experts in the health and fitness fields to begin focusing much of their efforts on getting people to move more rather than exercise more.

Some of the new recommendations coming out of this research hint that organizations such as the American Heart Association, the American Diabetes Association, and the American College of Sports Medicine should set a daily limit on sitting time. Many believe this limit should be no more than ninety minutes.

But can simply moving more really help with weight loss and be better than exercise? A study in the October 2005 issue of the journal *Chest* showed that jogging for twelve miles a week was not much different than walking for twelve miles a week from a weight loss perspective and that both dramatically enhanced cardiovascular health.

Some believe this effect is mediated by cortisol. Intense exercise releases more cortisol into the body, and this can have damaging effects. These effects seem to be mitigated by low-intensity movements like walking.

Walking allows you to move far more often without extra stress to your body and is one of the only forms of exercise that has been shown to lower cortisol and have a minimal impact on hunger. It also seems to be even more effective when done in a natural setting.

The take-home is that more exercise is not really that beneficial, but more movement is. You would be better off moving all day than sitting all day and then doing an intense bout of exercise. Walking lowers cortisol and does not stimulate the appetite.

That is why I recommend you try to get at least 10,000 steps per day. We are built to move, so do what you were made to do and get those steps in! Keep in mind that 5,000 steps is a little less than an hour a day for most people. If you shoot for two hours of walking, you'll be golden. Don't worry, this is not two hours at one time but rather total accumulated time walking around. A better way to measure this is to use a step counter. Two hours is about 10,000 accumulated steps during the day.

MEDITATION MATTERS

What do you think of when you hear the word "meditation"? If you're like many people, the word evokes the image of an utterly serene yogi sitting in a lotus pose under the billowing branches of a peaceful tree, all but levitating thanks to their unshakable focus. And for some people, that very well may be how they like to meditate. But the truth is, meditation is anything that allows us to get out of our own heads and into our own bodies. It's the thing you do that silences that inner voice saying, "How could that person do that to me?" or "Remember that awful thing that happened when I was a kid?" or "I'll never finish my to-do list!" Meditation is all about making that stress measurement on the metabolism barometer plummet down to zero.

Creative pursuits do a great job of forcing that voice to *shut up already*. Doodling, coloring, and playing musical instruments are just a few ways to lower stress hormones.

Surrounding yourself with greenery, particularly by taking a walk in nature, does the same thing (the Japanese even have their own word for being out in the woods, *shinrin-yoku*, which literally means "forest bathing"). Laughter is an amazing stress reducer, as is sex—the body's ability to orgasm is its own built-in stress-release function.

Anything that offers connection can be a form of meditation. This includes everything from lovemaking to simply spending time with people you care about, cuddling with pets, or engaging with your community. In this way, meditation can also combat one of the biggest stressors many people fear the most: loneliness. As a human, the feeling of being alone can be devastating. It's one of the reasons why heartbreak and loss of a loved one are so difficult. We all can benefit from a greater connection to humanity.

Exploring your unique purpose is another way to bring more peace to your life. This does not have to be some intense, overwhelming undertaking. Purpose is simply the humble recognition that you have certain signature strengths no one else has, and you can use those strengths to better the world. Understanding purpose anchors you and creates a force field against stress (more on this later).

BACK TO BASICS

The reason so many people are dealing with chronic stress and slogging through each day with a constant drain on their system is directly linked to the fact that we are not living in accordance with how we used to. We are ignoring the natural rhythms of our bodies. We think we can just keep ourselves in a state of perpetual stress and never experience a consequence. We don't stop to think about how the level of energy we expel determines the rest and recovery we need.

This boils down to basic math: if you're going to do an hour-long workout, you should plan for two hours of rest and recovery.

That can mean a relaxing walk or a short nap followed by some tai chi, or some time spent just listening to music or reading. Mindful metabolism masters know they have to be intentional about incorporating rest and relaxation into their schedules, perhaps even more so than they are about diet and exercise. It's easy to focus on what you're eating and how you're exercising. It's much more difficult for people to take a step back, look at themselves holistically, pinpoint their sources of stress, and actively work to address them.

Most people choose to continue living as if they're the one who's going to be plucked up at any moment by the pterodactyl. They become so familiar living with chronic stress that they never bother to pause, look around, and realize the terrifying creature is nowhere to be seen and most of the stress they're experiencing is self-created. Only shifting your focus from constant stress to improved mindfulness can help you see what's really going on, lower stress on your system, and help you keep everything in check.

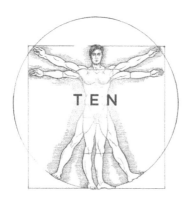

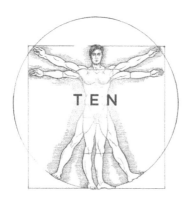TEN

THE METABOLIC
NUTRITIONIST

A s trends and fads continue to come in and out of our culture, you are still going to be bombarded with an array of different dietary approaches and corresponding gadgets. However, now that you are a metabolic detective, you will be able to view these with more context and scrutiny. Is this new approach simply ELEM in disguise? Is it ELEL? EMEM? You now have the knowledge to be able to strip each passing fad down to its basic metabolic toggle and determine if it offers any benefit to you and your unique makeup. You can do the same with new tech as it emerges. Any gadget that measures biometrics can be used as an adjunct to objectively gauging HEC and SHMEC. No new fad or product is going to stop your metabolism from constantly adapting, nor is it necessarily going to work with your own, individual physiology, psychology, personal preferences, or practical circumstances. The magic is in finding the tools that work best *for you*.

That being said, there are a few things you can add to your detective's tool kit that can offer additional insight into how your metabolism is working, what impacts it, and why.

KETO

When you don't have enough insulin in your body to shuttle glucose into your cells for energy, your body uses fat instead. Your liver takes that fat and converts it into ketones, which get sent into the bloodstream. We have the ability to measure ketones in the breath, urine, and blood as a means of determining how our body is burning fat.

As your body makes ketones primarily from fat and protein, fat burning ramps up. Once ketones start showing up in your breath, urine, and blood in high amounts, you know you are burning fat very efficiently. Ketones also are hunger suppressing.

Because of this, keto is an ELEL approach, similar to how hunter-gatherer humans lived when glucose was not always readily available. So although keto is an advanced technique, it also allows us to revisit a fat-burning state that was once very natural to us. When we were out in nature and only able to eat what we could grow or kill, we'd often spend the colder seasons existing on animal protein and small amounts of roughage. Our diet was mostly fat, some protein, and some fiber.

The keto diet calls for 70 percent or more fat with very little carbohydrates. Of course, everyone is going to differ slightly in their own individual needs, but in general, most people will reach ketosis by going below thirty grams of total carbohydrates per day. Some can hit ketosis at fifty or seventy-five grams. Regardless, it takes three to four days for ketosis to occur as your body uses up its stored glucose, and a warning: those first few days are going to be *rough*. Think of it like filling up your gas tank with diesel fuel when all you've ever used before is unleaded. That car is not going to run well at all. As your body switches over from running mostly on carbohydrates to burning up fat and creating ketones, you will experience what's known as "keto fog," or a few days of mental fatigue. But then, all of a sudden, your brain will come to life. Everything will start moving a little bit faster. You might start losing some weight. The benefits of the ketones will kick in, and you'll be on your way.

Contrary to popular belief, the keto diet is not that limiting. You'll be eating nearly all creamy, savory foods. When you wake up in the morning, you might have eggs and bacon with sliced avocado and tomato. Lunch could be salmon with a side of broccoli with plenty of butter, and a salad with cheese and ranch dressing. For a snack, you have a handful of nuts. For dinner, you might have steak with a side of greens. Then, if you have any allotment of carbohydrates left, you can have a cup of blueberries with some heavy whipping cream for dessert. Doesn't sound so bad, does it?

There are, however, some pitfalls of the diet. People who have eaten carb-heavy diets up to this point can struggle with the lack of starch. It also can be tricky to get those carbohydrates and proteins low enough, and if you don't, you never get into ketosis. You are never truly in ketosis unless you can measure ketones in your system.

There are three ways to measure ketones: in the breath as acetone, in the urine as acetyl acetate, and in the blood as beta-hydroxybutyrate. Most people who attempt keto make the mistake of only measuring ketones in the urine, which is not ideal because acetyl acetate peaks only in the beginning, then drops off. A better, and more accurate, approach is to measure in the blood and/or the breath (breath acetone correlates nicely with blood levels of eta hydroxy butyrate). The best way to do so is with a ketone meter, which you can buy online, at most pharmacies, and even at some local health food stores. It will require a finger prick, and the goal is to achieve a score of one to three on the meter. Measuring first thing in the morning is ideal because your ketones are highest after you've been fasting all night. As you become more aware of how your body is responding to the diet, you can start measuring after each meal. Your body constantly determines sugar levels and decides if it needs to make ketones, so the amount is always changing.

If you don't find ketones, *you are not in ketosis*. Instead, you are in AKZ—the almost keto zone—and likely feel terrible because you're not giving yourself the amount of sugar you're used to, but you also haven't ramped up ketone production. This is why measuring is so important.

Once you do get into ketosis, I don't recommend staying there for longer than three months. If you remain in ketosis longer than that, there is no danger, but as you have learned, it is best to switch things up from time to time to keep your metabolism flexible and responsive. Even four days is enough to get some of the benefits of ketosis. Ideally, I'd suggest staying in ketosis for at least a week and no longer than a few months at a time.

Keto falls under the ELEL toggle, so it's best done when you're not doing a great deal of physical activity. Even though ketones are known to be muscle sparing in their action, it is still possible to lose muscle just like with extreme ELEM regimes. After a period in ketosis, it helps to follow with an EMEM strategy so you can ramp up the carbs that will fuel your activity.

There are a lot of good keto alternative foods out there, but be warned: they don't work for everyone. On keto, you're getting a lot of very creamy, savory foods, and not much else. Some keto alternative foods tend to have artificial sweeteners, meaning some people who eat them are going to get more intense cravings for sweets. If this is you, following a pure keto approach with no alternatives will give you a better chance of success. A little bit of blueberry with some heavy cream is not going to mess with your cravings, but something like stevia might in some individuals.

Finally, when you end your keto diet, you should not follow it with a burger binge. Strong flavor hits aren't going to do you any favors. Instead, stick to relatively bland, protein-, fiber-, and water-heavy foods. Without those ketones in your system, you need to ramp up your major hunger-suppressing macronutrient, protein. Start with plenty of whey protein shakes, deskinned chicken breasts, and egg whites. Also, be aware of the halo effect that can hit after any diet. If you got good results on keto, you could be convinced that fat must not be that bad and want to keep more in your diet than you did previously. But you can't keep the fat as high as it was when you were pretty much *eating only fat*. When you're adding starch back in, you have to be aware of the balance you need moving forward. As carbohydrate intake swings back up, fat intake needs to come back down.

The keto diet has gained some popularity lately as research has shown its potential for helping with diseases associated with high blood glucose levels. It also jumped to the forefront when the CrossFit crowd discovered it a few years back.

It has come in and out of the spotlight, and although many people have reaped the benefits of it, it's also resulted in many failures (as do all diets). Most people fail simply because they are doing it wrong. For some, it's too restrictive based on the practical circumstances in which they live. That being said, people with easy access to fast food should find keto exceptionally easy to follow because you can have all the fatty meat you want.

Big Mac Attack

To keep starch low when eating fast food, all you have to do is ditch the bun and avoid the temptation of ordering a shake and fries with your burger. I wanted to prove this theory for myself, so for thirty days, I ate McDonald's every day while adhering to the keto guidelines.

I would order a Big Mac with extra lettuce, tomato, pickle, and onion. I'd leave the cheese and even add some bacon if I felt like it. Then I'd ditch the bun and put all of that on top of a side salad with a vinegar-based dressing. I dubbed this Jade's burger salad.

My results were phenomenal. I experienced weight loss and saw both my triglycerides and cholesterol go down. Granted, this diet is not ideal in terms of nutritional value, but it can actually be a fairly effective and healthy approach as long as it's not done for an extended period of time or repeated too frequently.

Prior to this experiment, I *hated* McDonald's. I was dreading getting started because even the idea of eating one greasy burger disgusted me. Now McDonald's is my go-to place when on keto. I love getting an Egg McMuffin minus the muffin, which is basically just eggs and cheese, and a black coffee. Or I get my burger salad and diet soda. I know I can order from the menu, make it my way, and stay on track.

You can do the same. If you find yourself with limited options, you can always make your own burger salad (or do a version of Dale's Slim Jim diet; remember him from earlier?). The bottom line is, you almost always have better options than what you might initially think.

INTERMITTENT FASTING

Another ideal approach to take after keto is intermittent fasting. Intermittent fasting is an ELEL toggle that works directly with the body's circadian rhythms. Humans are meant to have periods of time without food. Before electricity made it possible to stay up watching TV and snacking all evening, our meals were planned around the sun. We ate when it came up and stopped when it went down. Depending on the season, that meant we'd regularly go fourteen hours without food in our bodies, giving our digestive systems time to rest and clean up in a sense.

Imagine your body as a house where a never-ending party is happening. Music is blaring; people are coming and going. Until that party stops, there is no way you are going to get that house cleaned up. Everything just gets messier and more chaotic until eventually, things start to break. There are holes in the floor;

handles are falling off doors; windows are getting smashed. Before long, the house is a complete disaster. But if every once in a while, the party stops long enough for everyone to leave, you can get things in order. You can clean what needs cleaning and fix what needs fixing.

The way most of us live today is like subjecting our bodies to a never-ending house party. We never stop eating long enough for our system to reset. But by restricting feeding to specific times, our bodies are able to truly rest.

Intermittent fasting will look different for each person. For instance, you can't take someone who's used to eating from the time they wake up until the time they go to bed and expect them to go all day without food. That will make the metabolism more rigid. For most people, it's best to ease into it.

I suggest you start by going twelve hours without food. If you sleep eight hours a night, you need to avoid eating only a few hours before or after. If you want to make your metabolism even more flexible, simply extend that time frame by taking away either breakfast or dinner. Now you're moving into a sixteen-eight pattern, going sixteen hours without food and eight hours with it. Then you can extend it even further by taking away lunch and adopting an OMAD, or one-meal-a-day, approach. You can do an alternate day fast in which you fast for a day, then eat for the next one.

You can do a five-two approach, when you eat normally during the week and fast on the weekend. That doesn't mean you can't eat anything for two straight days. You can still get the benefits of fasting by staying under 500 calories a day. That means you can munch on celery, pepper, and other water-based, low-calorie foods and still adhere to your fast. You can have black coffee and chicken broth. You absolutely want to drink water to make sure you have some electrolytes. Then, during the week, you eat normally and healthily.

Regardless of the approach you take, it's key to remember there isn't anything magic about fasting. Even though you are creating a calorie deficit, you are not necessarily going to lose weight. It's just meant as a means to help the body clean itself out. People with extremely rigid metabolisms might actually see intermittent fasting backfire on them because it can lead to bingeing. Think of it this way: in natural settings, you would be hard-pressed to eat 2,000 calories a day. There simply wouldn't be enough access to calorie-rich foods like avocado, nuts, or honey.

However, in the modern day, you can easily consume 2,000, 3,000, 4,000, even 5,000 calories in just one meal. All it takes is one trip to the Cheesecake Factory. So for people who have trouble controlling their eating, intermittent fasting can be a slippery slope.

If you want to lose weight, you still have to have a calorie deficit and hormone balance. You can't fast, then binge, then fast, then binge the way many people do. You already know how to make sure fasting is working for you. Is it keeping HEC and SHMEC in check? If it is, it's working. As a result of skipping breakfast, do you eat more and worse at lunch and dinner? It's not working. Does skipping breakfast have no real effect on how you eat later? It's working. Again, there is no magic to it. It's just a question of whether it works for you.

As with keto, you don't want to break your fast with highly palatable foods that could send you on a binge. Always break your fast with large amounts of hunger-suppressing protein. If you're doing the five-two, your Monday and Tuesday meals should be somewhat bland. Also, as with keto, intense exercise does not work well with fasting. Walking, however, works perfectly well because it sensitizes the body to insulin, meaning you'll see a fat-burning effect. As an added bonus, it's a great way to get rid of some of the stress you might be feeling from not eating as much.

How long you decide to commit to a fasting cycle is up to you. For many people, it becomes embedded into their lifestyles. Then they are able to adapt and modify when need be. For instance, if you're on a five-two, weekday-weekend fast, but your family is having a huge get-together on Saturday and you know you'll want to indulge, you can adjust your fasting schedule. I come from a big Italian family that gets together and eats every Sunday—and boy, do we *eat*. In preparation, I fast all day Friday. Then, an hour before I meet up with the family, I lift weights. This way, I can essentially eat freely, and even if I overconsume, I know some of the calories are going to be used for repair.

Other times, I use a preload approach and eat something prior to the regular meal that will help offset calories. The best preloads are water-based, protein-based, and fiber-based foods that will fill you up and make you less likely to eat too much. A whey protein shake eaten thirty minutes prior to eating dinner might have 150 calories, but as a result of drinking it, you'll likely consume 400 less calories at the meal.

Intermittent fasting also can work well for women at specific points in their menstrual cycles. Women's temperatures change predictably right around ovulation, and monitoring devices such as the Daysy fertility monitor can tell them how to adjust their metabolic toggle based on their cycles to see the maximum benefits.

INTERMITTENT ENERGY RESTRICTION

Intermittent energy restriction is, at its most basic definition, a break from dieting. It's a prime example of the ESES toggle in action. Energy restriction for short periods of time makes the metabolism less compensatory. It's like a shock to the system that doesn't give the metabolism enough time to adapt or even create a severe stress response. The key is to do it long enough to get the effect, but not so long the metabolism becomes convinced it needs to regain all that fat.

There has been a great deal of research around the effectiveness of intermittent energy restriction, most notably the MATADOR (Minimizing Adaptive Thermogenesis and Deactivating Obesity Rebound) study, conducted in 2017. The study involved two groups: one that did two weeks of ELEL followed by two weeks of EMEM for thirty-two weeks, another that did two weeks of ELEL followed by two weeks of ESES for thirty-two weeks. Which group do you suspect saw better results—the group that had more exercise or the group that took regular breaks? The second group, or the people doing intermittent energy restriction, not only lost more fat, but they also saw less rebound weight gain.

Another study, known as the Scandinavian walking study, involved a group of men who did an extreme four-day diet for which they consumed only 300 calories per day but walked for nine hours daily across the Scandinavian countryside. In the end, each man had lost eleven pounds of fat. Over the course of the short study, they had created a daily 5,000-calorie deficit through continuous energy restriction. It was basically four days of extreme ELEM. Then they went back to a regular lifestyle of ELEL mixed with ESES. The most remarkable results, however, came a year later, when each person was still down at least four pounds of fat. I refer to the approach taken in this study as the reverse Thanksgiving effect because most of us in the Western world can easily gain four pounds of fat over Thanksgiving. We might lose two, but then we're still up two pounds from where we were before the holiday. Those two pounds stick around, then maybe we do the same thing at Christmas and end up wondering why we're ending the year heavier than we were last year. Do that for enough years in a row, and those pounds really start to add up. This study, however, was like a reverse Thanksgiving. By restricting their energy, even for a short period of time, the men were able to not only lose fat but keep it off long term.

All of these options are just a few examples of things you can try during your lifelong relationship with your metabolism to make it more resilient, more flexible, and more adaptable.

GLUCOSE DIETING

We covered this one briefly previously, but it is such an important concept and gives us huge clues as to what is to come regarding new approaches to being a metabolic detective that technology will be bringing us. Using biomarkers such as glucose has never been very practical up until recently. That is because all that was available was a snapshot in time. You stick your finger and you measure the sugar (glucose) concentration.

But what you could not know is if it had just risen to that number from a low place or just fallen to that level from a higher measurement. The only way you could practically get the full picture would be to stick yourself every few minutes and then graph the measurements.

New technology in the form of CGMs (continuous glucose monitors) does this for you. These devices contain a small probe that sticks into the skin, sampling blood from the capillary beds that perfuse the subcutaneous tissue. They also contain high-grade medical adhesives that keep the tracking device anchored into the skin. Once the unit is in, you don't feel a thing. It then, depending on the unit, automatically reads blood samples every couple of minutes and holds that data in the device. You can then use a reader or an app on your mobile device that downloads the accumulated data and graphs out your results. As long as you take a reading every six to eight hours, you will get hundreds of data points all at once (most of these devices store the data for only eight hours or so). Taking a reading only requires bringing your phone (or reader) close to the monitor.

You can then look back over the day and see when blood sugar spiked, when it crashed, and when it levels out. You'll know what it does when fasting, exercising, sleeping, and stressing, and most importantly, how it responds to certain foods. Recent research shows that our individual metabolic tendencies make themselves known when tracking glucose responses with certain foods.[40] One food in one person makes blood sugars spike. Give that same food to another person and you may see no spike at all or even a favorable response. You also get a sense of how poor sleep, lots of walking, cardio versus weights, or any other lifestyle factors interact with your ability to manage blood sugars.

Remember, the metabolism is always working to keep things in balance, and one of its most critical tasks is making sure blood sugar levels are not too high or too low.

To further understand this, let's go through a little of the science of blood sugar regulation, especially the concept of insulin resistance.

Insulin is the major hormone responsible for regulating blood sugar. Think of insulin like an arresting police officer. A prisoner is not just going to walk themselves to jail, in the same way sugar is not just going to jump into the cell. Insulin's job is to escort the sugar that's in the blood (blood glucose) into the cell where it can be processed for energy. Similarly, a riot where hundreds of criminals flood the street all at once means there is no possible way the police can handle all the criminals because they are spread too thin. Some of the cops may even be injured or killed and taken out of circulation if the riot gets too bad.

This is how to think about what happens when insulin is confronted with large amounts of sugar surges too frequently. It loses its ability to respond. This is what we call insulin resistance. The cells are no longer responding to insulin. It's like when you walk into a room with a strong smell. At first, you are aware of the scent and may even cover your nose. But soon, your sense of smell is downregulated and you are no longer aware of it. This is what happens with insulin.

The confusion for many people comes from the fact that insulin resistance is not all one thing. You can be resistant to insulin in one tissue and sensitive to insulin in another tissue. For example, when the liver is sensitive to insulin, it decreases glycogen breakdown and ramps up glycogen production (glycogen is how the body stores glucose away for a rainy day). The liver also shuts down gluconeogenesis (the body's own sugar-making process). After all, if enough sugar is coming into liver cells, it is prudent to use what is available, not raid your own pantry, and store excess for later use. You also would not bother yourself with needing to make anymore. However, if the liver becomes resistant to insulin, it continues to make new sugar and break down glycogen.

This means not only will you have blood sugar high from what you have eaten, but the liver will keep behaving as if you have low blood sugar and keep dumping sugar from its glycogen stores and making new sugar as well. This is like throwing kerosene and then gasoline on an already blazing fire.

The muscle too can be either sensitive to insulin or resistant. When muscles are sensitive to insulin, they suck blood sugar up like a sponge. Muscle uses this for the energy it needs to move around and also has the ability to store glycogen the way the liver does. The difference is that liver glycogen can be used to support the entire body, whereas muscle glycogen can only be used by the muscle and won't contribute to blood sugar levels. This tells you that when the muscle is resistant to insulin, glucose cannot get into the muscle and stays in the blood.

The brain and fat cells can also be either insulin sensitive or insulin resistant. In the brain, insulin acts as a hunger-suppressing hormone. If the brain becomes resistant to insulin, you will always feel hungry.

In fat cells, insulin increases fat storage and decreases fat release. So a resistant fat cell decreases fat storage and amplifies fat release. It is important to remember that fat release from fat cells (lipolysis) is not the same as fat burning (fat oxidation).

Many people have a ton of fat floating around in their bloodstreams that was released from fat cells that never gets burned and instead gets restored.

The law of metabolic individuality makes itself known here. People can vary in their sensitivity to insulin in different tissues. Genetics likely explains much of this. Being resistant to insulin at the level of the fat cell means that the individual is going to be leaner (less fat storage and more fat release). You might think that this would be a good thing, but all that fat has to go somewhere and it often finds its way into other organs instead, like the lining of the arteries.

This may be the reason we hear those stories of fit, lean-looking individuals dying of massive heart attacks in their forties or fifties. Insulin sensitivity in fat tissue may not make us look good, and it certainly is not healthy, but it may also keep us alive into our late sixties and early seventies as opposed to our late forties and early fifties.

This discussion of the different levels of insulin sensitivity in different tissues is required if you are going to understand how to use the new CGM devices now available.

If you wake up in the morning with high fasting blood sugar levels (i.e., >100), it likely means one of two things. It could mean you have an extra-sensitive stress hormone system that spikes cortisol and adrenaline levels in the morning. Cortisol is highest in the morning and this can explain why some people wake up with higher fasting blood sugars. Remember, you can stress your way into insulin resistance or eat your way there.

The other reason for fasting blood glucose in the morning is insulin resistance at the level of the liver. In this case, the background insulin signal is not being heard by the liver, so it continuously breaks down glycogen and makes glucose. This glucose then shows on your CGM as a high fasting blood glucose. This insulin resistance in the liver can be confirmed on eating. After a meal with sufficient carbs and/or protein, insulin levels should go up (fat by itself has very minimal to no impact on insulin). In a normal situation, blood sugar should rise and be near its highest around thirty minutes post-ingestion before falling back down to fasting levels within sixty to ninety minutes. A healthy response should not see the blood sugars go up much past 120 to 140 on the CGM. If, instead, the readings go up much higher, especially nearing 200, this is a sure sign the insulin sensitivity of the liver is compromised. By the way, in medicine, two first-morning fasting blood sugars of 126 or greater is diagnostic of diabetes. Being above 100 is considered prediabetic by many of us who practice integrative medicine.

The correct healthy response of a flexible insulin-sensitive liver should contain the degree of blood sugar rise. The blood sugars should then fall quickly within ninety minutes due to the sponge-like action of insulin-sensitive muscle tissue. This should look like a sharp peak when you see your glucose graph. If you instead see a plateau, when the glucose level stays high for longer than an hour, this is a sign that muscle insulin sensitivity is compromised as well. In this way, high fasting blood sugars as well as a very steep blood glucose rise signals issues with insulin at the liver. A blood sugar that fails to fall back down quickly may signal issues at the level of the muscle.

Once you understand these trends, you can start using your glucose monitor to track the beneficial effects of lifestyle choices.

For example, you will learn that exercise, especially intense exercise, will raise blood sugar similar to and sometimes greater than food. This is a stress response generated by the release of adrenaline and cortisol to provide fuel for exercise. You will then notice your blood sugars are on average lower and quicker to fall after eating in the hours and days after exercise. This is because exercise is a potent stimulator of the same glucose receptors triggered by insulin. In this way, contracting muscle circumvents insulin resistance of the muscle and is one of the best ways to restore proper blood sugar balance. Any type of exercise will do, but weight training may be best since there are some indications this form of activity can support liver insulin signaling as well.

Other things also work. Walking is a profound potentiator of this same muscle glucose receptor mechanism and also has a separate beneficial effect: the lowering of cortisol. Walking is so good at managing blood sugar because it simultaneously sensitizes the body to insulin while lowering cortisol. It also can be done for many hours without getting fatigued or overstressing the body.

You'll also learn which foods may be causing issues. You may discover that whole grain bread has minimal impact on blood sugar, but plain white rice sends your levels through the roof.

You may notice that steak and chicken included in a meal have different effects as well. Watching your blood sugar closely while monitoring your food intake teaches you lessons about your unique metabolic tendencies you could never learn otherwise.

Of course, blood sugar is not the only thing that matters. Just because your blood sugar levels look good on paper does not mean you can't store fat or are automatically burning fat. Calories matter too, and fat, which has the greatest number of calories per gram (nine compared to protein and carbs, which have four), does not have an appreciable impact on blood sugar. This is one of the reasons why adding fat to a sugary meal can blunt and slow the rise in blood sugar that follows. This can be beneficial for a diabetic who has uncontrolled high blood sugar levels but will do you no favors if you are trying to lose weight. When using glucose monitoring devices, you still need to attend to calories. However, using this tool along with close monitoring of HEC and SHMEC along with scrutinizing what you are eating and how what you are eating is impacting you gives you a huge amount of valuable information in finding what works and does not work for your unique physiology.

A couple of other points matter here. Insulin is a hunger-suppressing hormone both due to its impact on leptin and in its own right. Correlating blood sugar excursions based on what you are eating along with hunger in the hours after a meal tells you a lot about what will keep the brain happy and responsive to hunger cues.

There are also several different blood labs and vitals that you will want to pay attention to. High fasting blood sugars is one we have talked about, but lab tests can tell what's happening with blood fats as well. Fats don't float around the blood as single fats but rather as three fats bound to a glycerol molecule. This is called a triglyceride and is a direct measure of blood fats. When you see high fasting glucose and triglycerides, you can be assured that you are developing insulin resistance at the level of the liver muscle and/or fat cells.

This is a key laboratory measure of metabolic syndrome. When these two blood labs are elevated along with high blood pressure and a growing waist measure (a sign of visceral fat accumulation), this seals the diagnosis.

As things progress further, you may start seeing signs of liver distress as well. Alcohol abuse is a known cause of liver damage. However, those who have become insulin resistant in the liver start to accumulate the same kind of damage. It's called non-alcoholic steatohepatitis or NASH. This is a condition where fat starts to accumulate in the liver and liver cells become damaged. On your blood test, you will see elevations in one or more of the liver enzymes ALT, AST, and/or GGT.

Understanding the basics of what labs are telling you about your body gives you all the information you need to assess your individual metabolic flexibility. I recommend doing a full battery of basic blood labs quarterly in the beginning. There are many online direct-to-consumer labs you can use if your doctor is unable or unwilling to do these tests. Here is what to start with:

- *Complete metabolic panel with lipids and TSH.* This looks at the health and function of most organ systems and gives you total cholesterol and HDL and LDL as well as thyroid screening.

- *CBC with differential.* This looks at immune markers and screens for anemia.

- *Vitamin D.* This hormone is critical for multiple body functions.

- *Hemoglobin A1C.* This is a measure of average blood sugar for the last eight to twelve weeks.

- *Fasting insulin.* This number along with the blood glucose readings, hemoglobin A1C, triglycerides, and lipids will give you a good indication of how well your metabolism is functioning overall.

In addition, checking blood pressure regularly, weighing yourself, and measuring your waist circumference regularly (I recommend at least once per week) is essential.

All of this will give you invaluable insight into what your body is trying to tell you and what steps you can take to make sure you're allowing it to do what it needs to do to make your metabolism as healthy as possible.

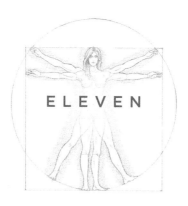

ELEVEN

METABOLIC
MAINTENANCE

Y ou now have all of the most advanced, up-to-date sci-
ence-backed information there is about metabolism.
You know why taking an individualistic approach to
and having a holistic view of your own unique metabolism matters. You know the power that comes with understanding
the very specific language your metabolism uses to communicate
with you every minute of every day. But having all this amazing
knowledge means absolutely nothing if you're ready to forget
every piece of it the first time things get hard.

You are, after all and above all, human. You are going to
encounter challenges. You are not immune to the ups and downs,
the frustrations and the follies all human beings are forced to deal

with on a regular basis. Remember that metabolism *does not give one single solitary damn* about what is or isn't convenient to you. It does not care about your time frame. It does not care about your desired outcomes. All it cares about—all it even knows how to do—is responding when it has something to respond to. You don't decide that you're doing everything right; your metabolism *lets you know* when you're doing everything right.

Metabolism is also a little bit crotchety. It's like an aggravated old man who's easily annoyed and thrown off course. Going on vacation can throw off metabolism. A stressful work week can irritate it. A few nights of restless sleep will do it. So will emotional turmoil. HEC, SHMEC, and even HRV will let you know when any of these things (or literally countless others) are pissing off your metabolism. It will give you a few small reactions before it actually smacks you in the face and forces you to take action. It's like that curmudgeon giving you a few strategically timed harrumphs before finally flipping you off.

You have to accept the fact that you are inevitably going to run into issues based on stages of life, stressful events, and many other factors. But the good news is that your metabolism and brain are working together in preparation for these rough patches by forming habits. Habits are shortcuts for metabolism, and it relies on these shortcuts whenever it gets overwhelmed or stressed. The bad news is, if you've developed some bad habits, there's no way to ever erase them. Instead, you have to replace them with new, better habits.

Habits happen in loops that become reminders, then routines, then rewards. One of my past clients was a perfect example of such a loop in action. Every evening after work, she would walk in the door, throw her keys on the counter, pour herself a glass of wine, cook dinner, turn on the TV, and proceed, over the course of the rest of the evening, to drink the rest of the bottle of wine.

Her reminder was simply walking in the door and tossing her keys down. Her routine was opening the wine, cooking, and turning on the TV. The reward was relaxation. We had to figure out a way to give her the reward without the negative routine.

I started by asking her about the things she loved to do to relax. She said she enjoyed taking walks with her husband, catching up with friends and family on the phone, and taking hot baths. Given that the first two options were dependent on other people, I opted to develop our plan around the baths. I told her to keep the step of tossing the keys on the counter. She even could pour that one glass of wine if she wanted. But before she started preparing her dinner, I told her to draw a bath, light some candles, and completely decompress.

Soon after implementing this plan, the benefits started to become apparent. Because she was delaying dinner, her husband had time to get home and start cooking some evenings, so now that responsibility was no longer solely hers. She did start out taking the bottle of wine to the bath but quickly realized the two did not mix and swapped the wine for herbal tea.

She still watched one episode of her show afterward but no longer found herself sitting in front of the TV for the remainder of the evening. Eventually, she even bought an infrared sauna, which took the place of the bath. She had completely revamped her reminder and routine habits, and the rewards were significant.

This is a perfect example of how simple it is to start swapping out old habits that no longer serve your goals with better behaviors that will get you closer to the results you want. You begin by reengineering the little things you do each day. Maybe you have a habit of lying in bed on your phone for an hour in the morning. Why not trade that time for a long, relaxing walk in the park? I encourage you to start looking for changes you can make, no matter how big or small. Try to find things that are similar or even easier than the things you're already doing but equally or more rewarding.

It also helps to know what triggers your bad habits. For example, many of us tend to turn straight to food the second we start to feel stress. It's our go-to comfort when we feel like things are spiraling out of our control. Yet, there are many other ways we can achieve a similar reward. We can get a manicure or pedicure; we can get a massage. We can masturbate or have sex—that might have made you blush, but the fact of the matter is, if you have an orgasm, you're not going to be thinking about cheesecake anymore. There is no shortage of enjoyable things that aren't food based that can deliver a similar sense of calm.

SEED STORIES

Oftentimes, our bad habits also can be traced back to our seed stories. These are our unique experiences that shape the way we view the world, and many of them are the exact reason why you eat the way you eat. Many of our seed stories are rooted in pain, and pain is capable of leading us to negative food-seeking behaviors.

But when you understand how your seed stories form your habits, you can also learn how to use that pain to empower yourself and make lasting positive changes.

We all have a "parents story" that impacts how we think about stability, safety, and love. Some of those stories might center on caring, stable environments where you felt supported and emotionally nourished. Some stories are far less ideal. Perhaps your parents story is rooted in uncertainty, fear, or sadness. In such cases, you might be turning to food to fill that void without even being aware of the cause of your behavior. In order to ever really change your habits, you will have to first change the way you handle that story. You might have to write your own story about loving yourself. Or you might have to replace the story with one about finding support outside the parent relationship. You can change it however you see fit, but until you do, that story will continue to shape and inform your choices.

We all also have a "child's story" linked to something that happened to you when you were young. Maybe you were teased like I was by my brother. For some people, that's not such a big deal. For me, it was torture. That story had the power to make me an angry person for a long time. It wasn't until I was in my twenties that I was finally able to step back and see that I was treating my brother more like the eight-year-old who used to pick on me than the man he had become. I had to rewrite that story, swapping out the jerk brother character for the guy who had become my friend. That changed how I viewed my brother as well as how I thought about all the other stressful things in my life.

The next story we all have is the "adolescent story," which is all about acceptance. This is the story that informs whether we believe we are attractive or ugly, well liked or unpopular, athletic or awkward, a "socially acceptable" size or too fat or too thin. The way we see ourselves as adolescents often follows us into adulthood, which is why we tend to compare ourselves to others instead of focusing on our own unique purpose.

The final story is the "adult story." This story shapes how we view loneliness, pain, and our responsibility over our lives and the decisions we make.

We all have to first take responsibility for our stories, then decide if we're going to use them to drag us down or lift us up. Pain can be a path to purpose but only if we are aware of it and in control of how we use it. For example, imagine you and I are in the kitchen cutting vegetables. If I slice my thumb, I will likely have a very predictable reaction. I will cover my thumb quickly, check to see how bad it's bleeding, clean the wound, and bandage it up. Then, the next time I'm cutting vegetables with you in the kitchen, I am going to be a little more careful. I might even look up videos on how to chop an onion correctly without cutting myself. I experienced pain, I learned from it, I grew, and I moved on.

However, if I was not prepared to handle pain, my reaction would be extremely different. I might get that same cut, then shove my thumb in your face, screaming that you need to do something about it. Or I might hide my hand behind my back and act like nothing is wrong. I might lose my thumb, but at least for now, I can pretend nothing ever happened. Maybe I'll just freeze up, stare at my bloody finger, and cry, ultimately doing nothing about it. These might seem like ridiculous options, yet these are the ways most of us handle emotional pain. We expect others to heal us. We hide it from others. We pretend it didn't happen. Not one of these methods is effective at healing any kind of pain or making it go away. The only way to begin to feel better is to acknowledge what happened and take responsibility for your role in making it better.

Planting New Seeds

The most effective way to gain power through pain is by conducting a story edit. This practice will help you convert a potentially draining, damaging seed story into a hero's journey.

Take out a notebook and write down *exactly* what happened as you remember it up until the present moment. This likely won't be easy. It might take some time. Don't feel the need to write perfectly or eloquently. Just get the story that has been hindering your growth, your progress, and your future down on the page, no matter how ugly it may be.

Next, write into the future explaining precisely how you will use that experience to propel you toward a place full of peace and fulfillment. Think about what that life would look like and describe it in intense detail. When you shed the weight of your past and pain and allow your mind to experience such a life, the path leading toward it becomes clear and you are able to see with clarity and focus.

In a sense, you are finishing the seed story, giving it new meaning, and exploring what the experience taught you. If this seems daunting or too complex for you wherever you are in your life right now, an even easier way to start is by identifying a similar pain in another person and helping them heal. Viewing pain through the eyes of an objective observer helps you gain perspective and rids you of any preconceived notions that have been stifling your own personal growth up to this point.

BUFFERS AND TRIGGERS

As you continue to explore your behavior and the reasons for it, you'll likely begin to recognize how unique your eating habits are, too. You can also write your food seed story to recognize and identify certain foods you turn to in specific scenarios. These foods fall into two categories—buffers and triggers—and every person has their own. Buffer foods are foods that, regardless of their health benefits, help you eat better and less. For example, you might be the kind of person who can have three Hershey's Kisses at 3:00 p.m. and, as a result, eat a salad with some grilled chicken at dinner and be totally satiated. That's a great balance—*if it works for you.*

For some people, having a glass of wine with dinner makes them less likely to have dessert. Other people will drink that same glass of wine at dinner, then need more and more wine, and dessert, and more food. For the first group, wine is a buffer food. For the second group, it's a trigger. Trigger foods are foods that, again regardless of health benefit, end up making you eat worse and more.

Your understanding of or assumptions about buffer and trigger foods is part of writing your food seed story. You likely believe certain foods are "bad" and certain foods are "good." But a handful of Hershey's Kisses that stop you from consuming an extra 500 calories is actually a health food. One glass of wine that leads to three more plus an order of chocolate volcano cake is pretty much the worst junk food you can consume. Similarly, if you're starving, one Snickers bar is good for you. If you've already consumed 5,000 calories in a day, any amount of broccoli or blueberries you eat is junk. You need to shift your thinking from "good" versus "bad" foods to foods that help you eat better and less versus foods that cause you to eat more and worse, regardless of what their health benefits are.

We've all been there. We might eat a small bowl of yogurt in the morning, a tiny salad at lunch, then plow through half a pizza for dinner. In this scenario, that yogurt and salad are not doing us any favors at all. All they are doing is triggering us to gorge later in the day. But maybe adding one spoonful of peanut butter in the afternoon might be enough to curb our cravings for the rest of the day. The peanut butter is a buffer, keeping us from overindulging and thereby undoing all the hard work we did all day.

Remember, as is the case with all things pertaining to metabolism, your buffer and trigger foods are different from everyone else's. Maybe you can't have just one spoonful of peanut butter—maybe one turns into two, turns into three, turns into half the jar. In that case, peanut butter is a trigger food for you.

But even though they are rarely the same from one person to the next, there are some commonalities. For most people, buffer foods are high in protein, fiber, and water and help them keep HEC and SHMEC in check for the longest intervals. Triggers are usually foods that combine sugar, salt, fat, and alcohol. These are generalizations, however, and only you can determine what foods help or hurt you the most.

To pinpoint your own buffer and trigger foods, simply think about what you eat and how it makes you feel. If you like wine, ask yourself if it helps you eat less or more. Do you casually sip a glass over an hour at dinner or do you throw back an entire bottle while simultaneously shoving a bag of chips into your mouth? Can you eat one piece of chocolate, or do even a few pieces send you on a bender usually reserved for small children on Easter or Halloween? Ask the same thing about peanut butter, cookies, yogurt, coffee, all of it. Make a list of both your buffer and trigger foods, and when you reach for one, ask yourself if it's going to offer you the most benefit in the long run.

BUFFER FOODS AND TRIGGER FOODS

Remember!
One person's buffer food can be another person's trigger food

COMMON BUFFER FOODS

Buffer foods help you eat less foods (and higher-quality foods) at future meals. Despite their calorie content or perceived unhealthy attributes, they lead to less food intake overall and a healthier, easier, more enjoyable diet.

- Cheese
- Chocolate
- Wine
- Bacon
- Sparkling soda
- Diet Coke
- Fruits
- Chewing gum
- Peanut butter
- Protein shakes

COMMON TRIGGER FOODS

Trigger foods cause you to crave the wrong foods and eat more of those and other foods at future meals. Despite their calorie load or perceived health benefits, they lead to a diet that is more fat-producing and less healthy overall.

- Doughnuts
- Chocolate
- Wine
- French fries
- Sparkling soda
- Diet Coke
- Pizza
- Sugar-free chewing gum
- Peanut butter
- Lettuce

Commit to Three

The best way to avoid trigger foods is to establish your three nutritional commitments. When life gets stressful and you revert to these habitual patterns, these three nutritional commitments will be your first aid kit. These are the three things that when you do them—and them alone—life is simple and easy. Again, they are unique to you. I can't tell you what yours are. You have to figure out what behaviors help you stay on track and make an attempt to commit to them each day.

My three nutritional commitments (which tend to work for most people) are:

- Eat my body weight in protein grams per day.
- Have two large salads per day.
- Drink four liters of water per day.

Easy, right? *Absolutely not.* I am never able to come close to consuming that amount of protein each day. In fact, if I hit two out of three commitments, I consider it a great day. Because even by doing just one of these three things, everything gets better. My HEC and SHMEC are in check, I'm less tempted by triggers, and I gain a sense of personal fulfillment. I encourage you to think of three similar things you can do that will anchor you when stressful situations arise and you're tempted to toss your focus on health and wellness goals out the window. These three nutritional commitments will give you focus, renew your dedication, and reaffirm your belief in yourself.

It also helps to have three lifestyle commitments, things you can do on a regular basis that neutralize stress and bring you back to center. Maybe you aim to have a regular massage, get eight hours of sleep per night, and take a long walk three times a week. Maybe you want to meditate for fifteen minutes every morning, turn off screens after 9:00 p.m., or check in with a supportive friend once a week. Those things act as a hormonal reset button for the body and become critical for combating the countless unforeseen stressors that will come your way.

3 NUTRITIONAL KEYSTONES

Choose 3 big nutritional habits that:

· Are easy to repeat day in and day out over months and years.

· Have large and beneficial trickle-down effects on hunger and calories.

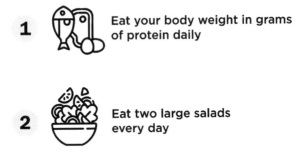

1 Eat your body weight in grams of protein daily

2 Eat two large salads every day

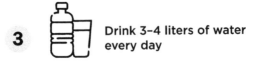

3 Drink 3–4 liters of water every day

When you have your nutritional and lifestyle commitments in place, stress can no longer threaten to derail your focus. You know that regardless of whatever challenge comes your way, you're going to have specific actions to fall back on. You might know you're facing a rough work week, but you also know you're going to have protein at every meal, which will keep you fueled and functioning at your best. Or maybe you're going to check in every week with your sister, who always gives you the best advice for navigating any situation. These commitments bring a consistency to your behavior that can't be shaken, no matter what uncertainty comes your way.

CONCLUSION

Human beings must constantly confront four certainties of life.

We all have to deal with loneliness. Even if we're regularly surrounded by other people, we all know deep down that ultimately, we are existentially alone.

We have to deal with freedom. The unlimited number of choices we face every day can overwhelm us and force us to settle because we know anytime we make one choice, we're forgoing something else.

We have to deal with meaninglessness. We can fabricate all the stories we want about why we are here, but the truth is, we don't really know.

Finally, we have to deal with death. Each one of us knows we have a limited amount of time to do whatever it is we believe we are here to do.

These four existential crises silently guide our lives every minute of every day. We might never intentionally think about them, but they are there, influencing every decision we make and every step we take. There are three ways most people deal with them, which I call the 3Ps: power, popularity, and—the only one that actually works—purpose.

We mistakenly believe that if we become powerful, we will never feel lonely, we will never struggle with freedom, we will never question our meaningfulness, and we will achieve some sense of immortality. But living only to chase power is the path to self-destruction. Power is often something you sacrifice everything to have, but it rarely, if ever, offers a return on investment.

We believe the validation of popularity will be enough to shield us from any pain or suffering. Yet, when we make popularity our sole mission, we actually end up losing our sense of self by trying to be who we think everyone else wants us to be.

The only way to deal with any existential crisis is by chasing purpose. Contrary to what you might think or what other books try to tell you, purpose is not complicated.

Purpose is simply the humble recognition that you are uniquely suited to offer something to the world that no one else can.

You have a unique voice. You have unique experiences. You have unique strengths as well as unique weaknesses. The stories that make up your life offer insight into what your purpose may be and how you can use it to contribute to the world around you. Your passion informs your purpose, as does your pain.

Your capacity to live a life of purpose is directly linked to your ability to be healthy, fit, and energetic, and there is no excuse to not want to be the best version of yourself possible in all areas. You have to have that solid foundation so when you do experience a setback, you can use your purpose to propel you past it.

When I ruminate about purpose, I always think about milk cartons. As a child of the 1980s, I can remember seeing the faces of missing children printed on those cartons. I'd stare at them every time I ate my cereal. I would always think about how the act of putting lost kids on containers of milk—a practice that saved the lives of thousands of people—likely started with one family. One child didn't come home one day, and instead of letting their pain debilitate them and dictate the course of the rest of their lives, those parents developed a solution to save others from the same fate. They turned their pain into purpose. Imagine what they had to do in an age when the internet wasn't even invented. They had to physically go to Congress to gain the attention and support of legislators. They had to appeal to the milk lobby. They couldn't stop because they were tired or overwhelmed or frustrated. They used their purpose to push their vision forward, and they never quit until it became a reality.

To live with purpose, you have to operate with the same level of energy, and the only way you do that is by committing to being as healthy as possible and listening to what your body is telling you. You have to link your ability to engage with your purpose to your own health and fitness journey, and you know by now what an important role metabolism plays in that.

This is what it truly means to be next level. To get there, you have to realize your own health and wellness are not just about you. It's not about vanity or power or popularity. Mastering your health and wellness is about your ability to do the things you want to do so you can make a positive impact on the world.

Early in my career, my brother and I were working as personal trainers at a gym in Seattle. One day, a significantly overweight woman came to us for help. As she spoke, she pointed to a poster on the wall behind me.

"See that woman?" she asked, gesturing to the before-and-after images of a person who was quite heavy in one and very lean in the other. "That's me."

The woman before me was even larger than the one in the before picture. She told me she had hit that goal weight once but was not able to sustain it.

I took her on as a client, and the first two years were a struggle. Her weight went down and up, down and back up, over and over until she finally hit a stretch where she was able to maintain a healthy weight for an extended stretch. I eventually asked her what had changed.

She told me she had watched a conversation between my brother and me that we had posted to YouTube. In it, my brother spoke about a study he had read that said children often adopt eating patterns similar to their parents'. We didn't know it at the time, but our client had an overweight daughter.

When she heard about that study, she knew she did not want her daughter to suffer a similar fate. If the daughter ended up emulating her mother, she'd struggle with weight her entire life. Our client knew she wanted the bad habits to stop with her. That was all the motivation she needed, and everything changed.

Whatever inspires your commitment to your own personal fitness, let it be rooted in purpose. It's not about getting a six-pack. It's not about fitting into a bikini. It's about taking your health to the next level so you are most able to share your unique gifts with the world.

ACKNOWLEDGMENTS

Thank you to Rachel LaBar for her amazing writing, direction, and instruction. Gratitude to Natalie Aboudaoud and the entire team at Scribe for their guidance and care. To my sister and personal assistant for always keeping me on track and having my back, thank you. To the millions of readers, followers, subscribers, podcasts listeners, patients, clients, professionals, and coaches who follow my work, do my workouts, and use these methods, thank you for your support, interest, and constructive feedback. You make this work possible.

NOTES

1   Katherine Hafekost et al., "Tackling Overweight and Obesity: Does
     the Public Health Message Match the Science?" *BMC Medicine* 11, no.
     41 (2013): PubMed 23414295; Traci Mann et al., "Medicare's Search for
     Effective Obesity Treatments: Diets Are Not the Answer," *American
     Psychologist* 62, no. 3 (2007): 220–33.

2   Catia Martins et al., "Metabolic Adaptation Is Associated with Less
     Weight and Fat Mass Loss in Response to Low-Energy Diets," *Nutrition
     & Metabolism* 18, no. 1 (2021): 60.

3   Erin Fothergill et al., "Persistent Metabolic Adaptation 6 Years after
     'The Biggest Loser' Competition," *Obesity* (Silver Spring) 24, no. 8 (2016):
     1612–19.

4   Ali Almajwal et al., "Energy Metabolism and Allocation in Selfish
     Immune System and Brain: A Beneficial Role of Insulin Resistance in
     Aging," *Food & Nutrition Sciences* 10, no. 1 (2019): 64–80.

5   Alison B. Evert and Marion J. Franz, "Why Weight Loss Maintenance
     Is Difficult," *Diabetes Spectrum* 30, no. 3 (2017): 153–56.

6   Catia Martins et al., "Metabolic Adaptation Is an Illusion, Only Present
     When Participants Are in Negative Energy Balance," *American Journal of
     Clinical Nutrition* 112, no. 5 (2020): 1212–18.

7   Kent Holtorf, "Thyroid Hormone Transport into Cellular Tissue,"
     Journal of Restorative Medicine 3, no. 1 (2014): 53–68.

8   Julie Calonne et al., "Reduced Skeletal Muscle Protein Turnover and
     Thyroid Hormone Metabolism in Adaptive Thermogenesis That

Facilitates Body Fat Recovery during Weight Regain," *Frontiers in Endocrinology* 10 (February 28, 2019): 119.

9   Mehmet Bolal et al., "The Relationship between Homocysteine and Autoimmune Subclinical Hypothyroidism," *International Journal of Medical Biochemistry* 3, no. 1 (2020): 1–7.

10   Maruizio Nordio and S. Basciani, "Myo-inositol plus Selenium Supplementation Restores Euthyroid State in Hashimoto's Patients with Subclinical Hypothyroidism," *European Review for Medical and Pharmacological Science* 21, no. S2 (2017): 51–59.

11   Candas Ercetin et al., "Impact of Photobiomodulation on T3/T4 Ratio and Quality of Life in Hashimoto Thyroiditis," *Photobiomodulation, Photomedicine, and Laser Surgery* 38, no. 7 (2020): 409–12; Yifang Hu et al., "Effect of Selenium on Thyroid Autoimmunity and Regulatory T cells in Patients with Hashimoto's Thyroiditis: A Prospective Randomized-Controlled Trial," *Clinical and Translational Science* 14, no. 4 (2021): 1390–1402.

12   Milind G. Watve and Chittaranjan S. Yajnik, "Evolutionary Origins of Insulin Resistance: A Behavioral Switch Hypothesis," *BMC Evolutionary Biology* 7 (April 2007): 61; Nicola Pannacciulli et al., "Anorexia nervosa Is Characterized by Increased Adiponectin Plasma Levels and Reduced Nonoxidative Glucose Metabolism," *Journal of Clinical Endocrinology of Metabolism* 88, no. 4 (2003): 1748–52; Saskia N. van der Crabben et al., "Prolonged Fasting Induces Peripheral Insulin Resistance, which Is Not Ameliorated by High-Dose Salicylate," *Journal of Clinical Endocrinology and Metabolism* 93, no. 2 (2008): 638–41.

13   Kimberly P. Kinzig, Mary Ann Honors, and Sara L. Hargrave, "Insulin Sensitivity and Glucose Tolerance Are Altered by Maintenance on a Ketogenic Diet," *Endocrinology* 151, no. 7 (2010): 3105–14; Gerald Grandl et al., "Short-term Feeding of a Ketogenic Diet Induces More Severe Hepatic Insulin Resistance than an Obesogenic High-Fat Diet," *Journal of Physiology* 596, no. 19 (2018): 4597–609; Michael Koffler and Eldad S. Kisch, "Starvation Diets and Very Low-Calorie Diets May Induce Insulin Resistance and Overt Diabetes Mellitus," *Journal of Diabetes and its Complications* 10, no. 2 (1996): 109–12.

14   Daniel Bunout and Gladys Barrera, "Seasonal Variation in Insulin Sensitivity in Healthy Elderly People," *Nutrition* 19, no. 4 (2003): 310–16.

15   E. M. Scott and P. J. Grant, "Neel Revisited: The Adipocyte, Seasonality and Type 2 Diabetes," *Diabetologia* 49 (July 2006): 1462–66; Peter J.

Grant, "Obesity, Adipocytes and Squirrels," *Diabetes and Vascular Disease Research* 1, no. 2 (2004): 67.

16 A. G. Unnikrishnan, "Tissue-Specific Insulin Resistance," *PMJ Online* 80 (2004): 435.

17 Keith N. Frayn, "Adipose Tissue and the Insulin Resistance Syndrome," *Proceedings of the Nutrition Society* 60, no. 3 (2001): 375–80; B. L. Wajchenberg et al., "Depot-specific Hormonal Characteristics of Subcutaneous and Visceral Adipose Tissue and Their Relation to the Metabolic Syndrome," *Hormonal Metabolism Research* 34 (November–December 2002): 616–21.

18 Keith N. Frayn, "Adipose Tissue as a Buffer for Daily Lipid Flux," *Diabetologia* 45, no. 9 (2002): 1201–10.

19 Sudha B. Biddinger and C. Ronald Kahn, "From Mice to Men: Insights into the Insulin Resistance Syndromes," *Annual Review of Physiology* 68, no. 1 (2006): 123–58.

20 Muhammad A. Abdul-Ghani et al., "Muscle and Liver Insulin Resistance Indexes Derived from the Oral Glucose Tolerance Test," *Diabetes Care* 30, no. 1 (2007): 89–94.

21 J. R. Daugaard et al., "Fiber Type-specific Expression of GLUT4 in Human Skeletal Muscle: Influence of Exercise Training," *Diabetes* 49, no. 7 (2000): 1092–95.

22 Yasuhiro Izumiya et al., "Fast/Glycolytic Muscle Fiber Growth Reduces Fat Mass and Improves Metabolic Parameters in Obese Mice," *Cell Metabolism* 7, no. 2 (2008): 159–72.

23 Ivan J. Vechetti Jr. et al., "Mechanical Overload-Induced Muscle-Derived Extracellular Vesicles Promote Adipose Tissue Lipolysis," *The FASEB Journal* 35, no. 6 (2021).

24 Dori M. Steinberg et al., "Weighing Every Day Matters: Daily Weighing Improves Weight Loss and Adoption of Weight Control Behaviors," *Journal of the Academy of Nutrition and Dietetics* 115, no. 4 (2015): 511–18.

25 Suzanne Phelan et al., "Behavioral and Psychological Strategies of Long-Term Weight Loss Maintainers in a Widely Available Weight Management Program," *Obesity* 28, no. 2 (2020): 421–28.

26 N. M. Byrne et al., "Intermittent Energy Restriction Improves Weight Loss Efficiency in Obese Men: The MATADOR Study," *International Journal of Obesity* 42, no. 2 (2018): 129–38.

27 Christopher B. Scott, Alicia Croteau, and Tyler Ravlo, "Energy Expenditure before, during, and after the Bench Press," *Journal of Strength and Conditioning Research* 23, no. 2 (2009): 611–18.

28 Christopher B. Scott, "Contributions of Anaerobic Energy Expenditure to Whole Body Thermogenesis," *Nutrition & Metabolism* 2, no. 14 (2005).

29 Mark D. Schuenke, Richard P. Mikat, and Jeffrey M. McBride, "Effect of an Acute Period of Resistance Exercise on Excess Post-exercise Oxygen Consumption: Implications for Body Mass Management," *European Journal of Applied Physiology* 86, no. 5 (2002): 411–17.

30 E. G. Trapp et al., "The Effects of High-Intensity Intermittent Exercise Training on Fat Loss and Fasting Insulin Levels of Young Women," *International Journal of Obesity* 32, no. 4 (2008): 684–91.

31 Edward L. Deci and Maarten Vansteenkiste, "Self-determination Theory and Basic Need Satisfaction: Understanding Human Development in Positive Psychology," *Ricerche di Psicologia* 27, no. 1 (2004): 17–34.

32 Panteleimon Ekkekakis, "Let Them Roam Free? Physiological and Psychological Evidence for the Potential of Self-selected Exercise Intensity in Public Health," *Sports Medicine* 39, no. 10 (2009): 857–88.

33 Andrew M. Edwards et al., "Self-pacing in Interval Training: A Teleoanticipatory Approach," *Psychophysiology* 48, no. 1 (2011): 136–41.

34 Ekkekakis, "Let Them Roam Free?" 857–88.

35 Lindsay R. Duncan et al., "Exercise Motivation: A Cross-sectional Analysis Examining Its Relationships with Frequency, Intensity, and Duration of Exercise," *International Journal of Behavioral Nutrition and Physical Activity* 7, no. 7 (2010).

36 Edwards et al., "Self-pacing in Interval Training," 136–41.

37 Habil Hamdouni et al., "Effect of Three Fitness Programs on Strength, Speed, Flexibility and Muscle Power on Sedentary Subjects," *Journal of Sports Medicine and Physical Fitness* (February 2021).

38 Norman Pecoraro et al., "From Malthus to Motive: How the HPA Axis Engineers the Phenotype, Yoking Needs to Wants," *Progress in Neurobiology* 79, nos. 5–6 (2006): 247–340.

39 Joseph Henson et al., "Associations of Objectively Measured Sedentary Behaviour and Physical Activity with Markers of Cardiometabolic Health," *Diabetologia* 56 no. 5 (2013): 1012–20.

40 Patrick Wyatt et al., "Postprandial Glycemic Dips Predict Appetite and Energy Intake in Healthy Individuals," *Nature Metabolism* 3, no. 4 (2021): 523–29.

ABOUT THE AUTHOR

Before reaching millions of people worldwide with his workout videos and books, Dr. Jade Teta was a personal trainer for twenty-five years. He is what his friends describe as part science nerd, nature boy, jock, and philosopher. He holds a degree in biochemistry, a doctorate in natural medicine, is working on his PhD in clinical psychology, and is a licensed physician specializing in functional endocrinology (the study of hormones). His expertise spans three main areas: mindset, muscle, and metabolism. He publishes books and creates programs in two genres—physical development and personal development. His two greatest passions are working out and writing, as evident by the many books he has authored focused on helping people reach and maintain their health and wellness goals, as well as their aspirations in purpose and meaning. He is the founder and creator of Next Level Human and part owner of *Metabolic.com*. Learn more at *jadeteta.com*.